Heal From Within: Your Essential Guide To Natural Remedies and Holistic Medicine

Achieve Quality of Life Without Pharmaceuticals, Ease Anxiety, Boost Immunity, And Reduce Chronic Pain

James Mercer

Table of Contents

Introduction

In the whirlwind of our daily lives, where responsibilities pull us in every direction, our personal well-being often gets lost in the shuffle. The weight of these demands, both physical and emotional, takes a toll on our health. Balancing our daily obligations with our own health needs leads us to search for alternatives beyond the usual medical choices such as reliance on pills. This book is an invitation, guiding you toward a new path of self-healing and showing you how to reclaim control over your health choices.

This book is a roadmap, with the intent to empower and uplift you by revealing the intricate connections between our mind, body, and the natural world—which is essential for creating a life of balance and resilience.

At the heart of our exploration remains the goal of self-care—an unwavering belief in our ability to shape our well-being by seeking holistic solutions and embracing the power of self-healing.

Modern healthcare has benefited from some wonderful discoveries and developments over the last 150 years, including vaccines, x-rays, chemotherapy, and a multitude of other new techniques for diagnosing and treating illnesses and diseases. However, the ways in which we have used some of these medicines have created new problems. Antibiotics have now been over-used so much that some bacteria have evolved to resist their effects, creating superbugs like MRSA that can't be treated. Over-the-counter medicines are being used to treat symptoms and leave the underlying problems unaddressed. Sometimes we're even guilty of stacking medications by taking something to relieve the side effects of another pharmaceutical drug. How have we ended up with a medical system where treatments can make us feel worse instead of better?

You might have read headlines stating that the number of cases of diseases like cancer and diabetes is on the rise. The fact is that they have been steadily climbing for years, and so has the amount of money that healthcare providers have to spend to deal with them. It is predicted that between 2022 and 2027, spending on oncology treatments will hit an annual growth rate of 16%, spending on immune diseases and diabetes will see an annual growth rate of 6%, and spending on treatments for obesity will balloon by 38% each year.

What do all these diseases have in common, apart from their increasing prevalence? They're not caused by viruses or bacteria, you can't catch them from someone else, and you can't pass them on. No, these medical issues are caused by our modern lifestyle: living in polluted cities, eating processed and sugary foods, and pushing our minds and bodies to the limit.

When Medication Becomes Unnecessary

By using pharmaceutical drugs to treat the symptoms of a condition like diabetes or high blood pressure, doctors are giving the illusion of making a difference when really they're only masking the problem. This is typical of modern medicine, which relies on an allopathic philosophy—treating the symptoms to make the patient feel better, rather than looking at other ways to stop the symptoms from occurring in the first place. Traditional medicine takes a more holistic approach—treating the whole person and using their symptoms to point toward areas where they need to make changes.

Here's a simple example of how both systems work. A patient presents with high blood pressure and the allopathic response is to prescribe ACE inhibitors. These lower his blood pressure but he suffers side effects including nausea and headaches, which he treats with antiemetics and painkillers. The holistic treatment recognizes that high blood pressure is usually caused by lifestyle factors such as being overweight, having an unhealthy diet, and not exercising enough. Cutting out salty and fatty foods, reducing caffeine and alcohol, and adding three moderate exercise sessions a week reduces his blood pressure without the need for medication and with no side effects.

So, why is prescription medication usually the first response when there are cheaper and healthier treatment options for many of the most common health complaints? There is a perceived view in society that they work faster and are easier than making lasting lifestyle changes, and to some extent that is correct. However, in the long run, these changes can have a much wider benefit and prevent you from developing further conditions and diseases in the future. You might need to take medication to address an immediate and urgent problem, but by following up with gradual, small lifestyle adjustments, you may not need to be on that medication for the long term.

Cara's Story

Cara struggled with depression and anxiety as a teenager and was prescribed Prozac to treat it. She tried a couple of times to come off the medication in her early twenties, but each time the depression and anxiety returned and she had to restart the prescription. She doesn't like the way Prozac makes her feel; she suffers from digestive discomfort and diarrhea that she needs to take other medication for, and her head always feels a little fuzzy. Cara has been taking Prozac on prescription for ten years now.

Last year, Cara moved to a new city and started seeing a different doctor. She mentioned that she would like to try coming off the Prozac again and explained the problems she'd had in the past. The doctor recommended a series of Cognitive Behavioral Therapy (CBT) sessions with a trained therapist and also sent Cara to see an herbalist. The CBT helped Cara learn some ways to manage her anxiety and depression, including using meditation and visualization to anticipate the outcomes of stressful events. Cara also started swimming regularly, as she found that being in the water gave her time to think through the events of the day and let go of any unhelpful thoughts. The herbalist recommended Cara start taking an extract of ashwagandha to replace Prozac, as it has a similar effect but without unwelcome side effects.

When she only treated the symptoms of her anxiety and depression by taking Prozac, Cara wasn't doing anything to investigate why she felt that way. By learning to redirect the anxious thoughts and not obsess over the ways things could go wrong, her levels of anxiety were reduced and she didn't need medication to control them anymore. She finally felt like she was more in control of her life, which helped to improve her mood and reduce her feelings of depression. For the first time in ten years, Cara is off prescription medication and not having to deal with the side effects, making her life more uncomfortable.

Complementary Treatments

Within these pages, we're going to explore some of the many complementary treatments that take a more holistic approach to healing. Some of these can be used alongside modern medicines and others are able to replace them completely. It all depends on what you're trying to treat. I'm not here to tell you that the right combination of herbal teas will be as effective as chemotherapy for treating cancer, but they can reduce some of the side effects and help you feel less tired.

You should always discuss this with your doctor or another qualified medical professional if you're considering seeking complementary or alternative therapies. They might be able to recommend someone for you to see, or they could advise you about which are the most appropriate to look into. Most doctors nowadays have seen the benefits of complementary therapies, and there have been hundreds of research studies that back up their claims with solid results. Keeping your doctor informed of all your treatments is important so that they can avoid prescribing you something that will work against another therapy.

It's also worth noting that the FDA does not approve any herbal treatments or standardized doses. You'll see this warning printed on the packets of herbs you can buy. It doesn't mean that they aren't safe or effective, just that the FDA has not put any rules in place to regulate the industry.

1. The Power of Holism

In order to decide how to make holistic medicine work for you, you need to know more about where it comes from. In this chapter, we'll look into some of the key tenets of holism as well as dive into the history of some of the oldest forms of traditional medicine that still influence complementary therapies today.

The Holistic View of Health

Holism considers all aspects of a person's life and looks at ways they can make lasting changes that will improve their health. Instead of giving you pills to simply make your headache go away, a holistic practitioner would try to understand what is causing the headache in the first place. Are you dehydrated, stressed about something, overtired, or eating badly? All of these can cause headaches and most are easy to fix without needing medication. If you treat a symptom holistically, you have a greater chance of it not recurring because the underlying problem will be solved.

Modern medicine separates you into smaller and smaller categories when trying to find a way to help. The first way they do this is by determining whether your problem is physical, emotional, or psychological/spiritual. Holistic medicine understands that these aspects of you are intertwined and it's always better to look at the bigger picture. If you're feeling anxious (emotional pain), it affects you physically—you feel sick, your hands shake, and your vision gets blurry—because you can't simply divide your illnesses, diseases, and conditions into nice, clean categories.

It's not surprising that more people are turning to holistic medicine. Our lives are getting more hectic and stressful and modern medicine isn't helping as much as we thought it would. Holistic practices have helped people for thousands of years, long before we had problems with processed food, nicotine addiction, not getting enough sunlight, or bad posture from sitting at desks all day. Using ancient healing techniques can help us escape from the disadvantages of the modern world and remind us of our connection with nature, the universe, and all parts of ourselves.

Mind-Body-Spirit

The ultimate goal of holistic healing is to balance the mind-body-spirit connection and unify all aspects of our health. Mind refers to your thoughts, emotions, and feelings, and when it is strong, you'll feel confident, clear, and focused. Body refers to your physical self and all aspects of physical health and fitness. Spirit doesn't have anything to do with your religious identity, instead, it means your connections with people and with nature, intentions, and goals, and how you fit into the world around you.

If one part of this connection is troubled, it will show symptoms in the others. Many people struggle most with their spiritual side, and while you can take pills to treat the physical and mental problems that arise from this, they do nothing to attend to the problem itself. We live in a world where it's difficult to take time for ourselves, to slow things down and consider who we are and what we're doing. Forging connections with others has become harder because we often don't have the time or energy to invest in fledgling relationships. We're discouraged from doing nothing, even if that nothing is spiritually refreshing.

Ancient Holist Practices

There isn't just one form of holism; rather, different cultures have each developed their own distinct style of treating people. We can trace rituals, herbal medicines, and other treatments back thousands of years and many of their cures and claims have since been proven by modern science. The oldest forms of holism still practiced today are Ayurveda—from India—and Traditional Chinese Medicine (TCM).

Most ancient medical systems tried to explain illness as an imbalance or disruption of a spiritual part of you that couldn't be seen. Remember, we didn't know about germ theory—the viruses and bacteria that cause infections and make us ill—or genes and how they affect our bodies until the 19th century. Ancient doctors and scientists needed a way to show that your symptoms were a sign of something wrong, even if they didn't know exactly what caused them. So, while these theories aren't supported by modern science, quite a lot of the links they make are surprisingly sound. For example, in Ayurvedic medicine, swelling and inflammation in the joints were linked to having too much heat energy and were treated by applying cooling salves and drinking cooling teas, the theory being that cold energy would balance the excess heat. It worked, and it still works, even if the explanation for why it does has changed.

Ayurveda

The oldest Ayurvedic texts date back to 3000 BCE, but they were being practiced before then with the philosophies and remedies passed down by word of mouth. Ayurveda seeks to help you achieve balance and strengthen your connections, both internally between the body, mind, and spirit and externally with nature and the cosmos. This philosophy was one of the first to recognize that how we live our lives can disrupt the natural balance, and it urges people to make conscious choices to readdress these disturbances through meditation, nutrition, and yoga.

Ayurvedic practitioners identified a number of different elements and qualities that make up your constitution, known as your *prakturi*. Your *prakturi* consists of three *doshas* that are influenced by different elements: *pitta* is the fire element and controls your digestive system and your perception of the world; *vata* is ruled by the elements space and air and it controls your creativity and comprehension, and *kapha*, ruled by earth and water, which promotes self-healing and positive emotions.

This holistic approach balances curative medicine with a preventative approach, believing that it is better to maintain your health than to try and fix it. Ayurvedic practitioners have been recommended by doctors to help manage the side effects of patients undergoing cancer treatments or who suffer from chronic conditions. They do this by designing nutrition, exercise, and meditation regimes and introducing boosting herbs like neem (detoxifies blood), shatavari (digestive issues), and ashwagandha (immune system).

TCM

Like Ayurveda, TCM also has its origins over 5,000 years ago, and today we use several of its treatments as complementary therapies, including acupuncture, cupping, massage, and herbal remedies. At its core is the belief that we all have an invisible life force called Qi that is balanced by two opposing influences called yin and yang. An imbalance in your Qi, caused by too much yin or yang, would bring about an illness that could only be treated by restoring the balance.

Practitioners also believed that your body was influenced by the external elements: Earth, fire, water, metal, and wood. Too much of one of these elements would also affect the balance of your Qi. There are a number of different ways to restore balance, including physical treatments and herbal medications you could take.

Acupuncture and cupping were designed to break up blockages that stopped your life force from flowing freely. Practicing Tai Chi will help to strengthen the connection between your mind and your body and teach you to focus on balancing your Qi. Herbal medicines can be taken to treat a specific symptom, like jujube seed, which is a natural sedative that calms anxiety, or as a tonic to achieve and maintain balance, like astragalus root, which boosts your immune response.

Western Herbalism

The first records of Western herbalism come from the Ancient Greeks and Romans around 400 BCE. They collected treatments, plants, and information from all the countries they invaded, like scientists collating their research from different projects. These herbal cures formed the basis of Western medicine for hundreds of years. Unlike Eastern holistic practices, Western herbalism treated illnesses as symptoms of something physically wrong, trying to move away from theories that you were sick because you'd been cursed or had sinned.

Western Herbalism has the most comprehensive library of herbal treatments because it took information from sources all over Europe, Africa, and Asia. In the 10th century, the medical university at Salerno, Italy, became the first place to transcribe medical texts from Arabic and these provided even more information about plants and their uses. Then, in the 16th century, printing presses brought herbal cures to the masses and people started to keep their own apothecaries at home.

Many common herbal remedies that are used today have been around for thousands of years, like drinking calendula tea for an upset stomach or rubbing witch hazel on bee stings. Even pharmaceutical drugs like aspirin and several chemotherapy treatments have been inspired by the properties of plants.

Other Herbal and Holistic Therapies

Herbalism was the main form of medicine all over the world until the middle of the 19th century. Native American tribes used local herbs in many of their spiritual rituals as well as to treat physical ailments. The same is true for Aboriginal Australian, South American, and African medicine. Each of these also speaks about a link between your physical health and your spiritual health and how one couldn't be healthy if the other wasn't. Using local plants was very important and different tribes would share their knowledge so herbal cures were spread by word of mouth.

When invaders came from other lands, like Spain, England, France, and Italy, they took some of the plants back home with them and added to the herbalist knowledge in their own countries.

Some of these plants became naturalized and started to grow in the wild, while others were specially grown in medicinal gardens. Increasing access to a wider range of herbs meant that better cures were more readily available all over the world.

Modern Medicine

There isn't an exact moment that can be hailed as the birth of modern medicine and the shedding of old ideas, but the 19th century was full of new medical discoveries like x-rays, antibiotics, and vaccinations. As technology developed, doctors and scientists invented new ways of diagnosing and treating illnesses, including improved surgical techniques and mass-produced medicine. Some medicines use extracts from plants, building on the knowledge that has been passed down for thousands of years, but not necessarily making the treatments more effective. In fact, there have been scientific studies to show that isolating and taking just one part of a plant actually makes the treatment less effective (Karimi et al., 2015).

At some point, we began to trust modern medicine more than thousands of years of herbalism and holistic healing. Maybe it's the allure of science and the view that all new technologies and developments are designed to improve our lives. After all, surely the doctors know more than your Aunt Janice and her hippy friends?

Key Philosophies

Although different medical systems developed all over the world they have a surprising number of core beliefs in common. The main one is an agreement that your overall wellness is multifaceted and you need to pay equal attention to all different areas. These have been called the **Four Pillars of Holistic Well-**

ness and they are physical, mental, emotional, and spiritual health.

- Physical health isn't just about not being sick, it also means taking care of your body, both inside and out. Getting enough sleep, exercising regularly, and eating a balanced diet are all important parts of making sure you're physically well, as is avoiding excessive amounts of alcohol, cigarettes, and other harmful substances. Feeling physically unwell is often the first sign that something is out of balance because it's the best way your body has to communicate its needs to you.
- Mental health has the ability to process everything that happens in your day, to be able to focus on the tasks you need to complete, and to know how to relax and wind down at the end of the day. This can be helped by meditation and calming exercises like yoga and tai chi, but also by making time to do things you enjoy, spending time with friends, and making sure you set clear boundaries in your work life so you aren't taking on too much stress.
- Emotional health is all about processing your feelings and emotions in a healthy manner. It's not being happy all the time, but rather accepting when negative emotions come along and finding ways to either channel them productively or know how to diffuse them. Journaling can help you recognize how you respond to different emotions, and talking with a therapist or trusted friends makes sure bad feelings don't get bottled up and turn into something worse.

- Spiritual health is not about following a religious path, but following a path that is true to you and finding your direction. Think about your values and what you consider important in your life. If you spend time devoted to these things, you'll experience spiritual wellness, but if you don't, you can start to feel worthless or directionless. Spending time in nature can help you feel connected to the universe and give you a better sense of where you fit into the grand scheme of things, as can prayer and meditation.

Holistic therapies work by helping you identify which of these pillars you've been neglecting and working with you to find ways to refocus some of your time and attention on healing them. Sometimes, it's a quick fix, like fitting in an exercise class once a week or swapping your regular coffee for decaf. Other times, it might take longer, especially if you need to look inward and discover what really makes you happy.

Backed Up by Science

In the last decade, doctors have started to return to more holistic practices in order to help their patients receive the best treatment. Known as complementary therapies, these treatments are not recommended as a replacement for modern medicine, but to work alongside the plan prescribed by your doctor. A lot of research has gone into how these complementary therapies can help boost recovery rates, increase patient comfort, and reduce the side effects of pharmaceutical drugs.

Holistic medicine is all about treating the whole person, attending to each of those four pillars mentioned above, and that includes using modern medical treatments to heal the mental and physical aspects of an illness. However, using complementary therapies gives practitioners a much larger toolbox to draw from when considering how best to treat their patients. If someone is suffering side effects from their prescribed treatment, do you offer them more drugs or send them to an herbalist for something a bit gentler? Someone who is finding it difficult to cope with the mental and emotional effects of having major surgery could be prescribed antidepressants or they could talk to a therapist or practice meditation to process their thoughts. You have the right to choose your options.

John's Story

John was diagnosed with Hodgkin lymphoma in 2021 and his consultant recommended a course of chemotherapy. After a few sessions, John began to feel tired all the time. He lost his appetite, felt nauseous, and found it difficult to eat because his mouth was sore. He spoke to his doctor, who recommended painkillers and anti-sickness tablets. The anti-sickness tablets caused more side effects, this time constipation and headaches. John began to feel like he couldn't continue with the chemotherapy, even though he knew it was his best chance of beating cancer.

Fed up with feeling miserable, John went back to his doctor and asked if there was an alternative to the tablets, as they were making him feel so much worse. She sent him to speak to a holistic practitioner who specializes in helping cancer patients manage their symptoms and side effects of the treatment. Together, they designed a program that John felt comfortable trying. It included acupuncture to help with nausea and a gentle exercise program of yoga and short walks to help with the fatigue.

John's holistic doctor also introduced him to a nutritionist. She advised him on which foods were easy to digest and recommended he start drinking chamomile tea to help relieve his sore mouth.

After two weeks, John felt more energized and was able to eat without pain or nausea. He finished his course of chemotherapy and has been in remission ever since. He kept up the yoga because he enjoyed it and found it also lifted his mood, but he was happy to stop drinking the chamomile tea as he much preferred his regular cappuccino.

2. Listening to Your Body

One of the most important things holistic therapies can teach you is how to check in with your body. This is your way of having a conversation with yourself and seeing if your body can give you any clues that let you know something needs your attention. You might think it would be easy, it is your body after all, but you'd be surprised how bad we all are at listening to what it tells us. Would you be able to recognize whether your headache was caused by stress, overstimulation, illness, or a stiff neck? Each one feels slightly different, but unless you're taught to read the signs, you might just take some aspirin and wish it away.

Reading Body Language

Your body has a couple of different ways of responding to illnesses and issues. If it's battling an infection, the immune system response will kick into action, but if it's a mental or emotional issue, it will trigger a stress response. Understanding how both work will help you better recognize what is making you feel unwell or off-kilter.

The Immune System

Your immune system is your body's defense against invading microbes like viruses and bacteria. The most important parts are your white blood cells and antibodies. When they find microbes in your body, they send messages to the rest of your immune system to start destroying them. Sometimes these microbes can make you feel ill, like a viral infection in your throat that makes it sore, but other times the symptoms you experience are actually caused by your own immune response. Good examples of these are a fever—your body raises its own temperature to kill off bacteria—and a cough—your body tries to expel invading microbes.

When you have a raised temperature, do you automatically reach for medication to reduce it? According to Geddes (2020), this might not be a good thing. For most people, having a slightly raised temperature can be beneficial because it helps their immune system work more effectively. Unless you have an existing heart condition or your fever reaches 104°F, you could be doing more harm than good by trying to bring your temperature back to normal.

A Helpful Stress Response

When we talk about stress, it's usually cast in a bad light. Too much stress can be very bad for you, but in small doses, stress is your body's way of helping you focus and power through a difficult situation. When you are put in a difficult situation, for example, if you have a looming deadline at work or you're having dinner with your in-laws, your brain triggers a chemical response to try and keep you safe. This is often known as the "fight-or-flight" response because it prepares your body to either power up and battle the source of your stress or run away from it. It's this response that gives you a second wind when you're having to work late or makes you want to run and hide if you hear your boss on the rampage.

When you go into "fight-or-flight" mode, you'll notice some very obvious changes in your body. Your heart will start to beat faster and your breathing will become quicker and more shallow. Your muscles tighten and you might find that you're clenching your jaw or scrunching your hands into fists, or you could start fidgeting, bouncing your knee up and down, or pacing the room. This is because you now have more adrenaline in your body and it's keeping you ready for action, like a tensely coiled spring. This is great if you're about to run into a burning building or away from a hungry bear—and once you're finished fighting or fleeing, your body chemistry, and the changes it caused return to normal—but if you don't actually do anything as a result of this heightened stress, your body stays in this state, and that can cause its own problems.

Why De-Stressing is Important

Long-term stress not only feels extremely uncomfortable but it can have a real physical effect on your body. Think how quickly your car's engine will burn out if you keep revving it all the time, or how soon you'll wear down a pair of new shoes if you keep stepping in them even when you're sitting down for hours. This is exactly how your body feels when it spends too long in "fight-or-flight" mode; being constantly ready for something to happen will cause you to wear out quickly, both emotionally and physically.

Spotting Symptoms of Stress

Everyone deals with stress differently. Some people can handle a lot before they start to feel unwell but others find it extremely difficult to cope with even the slightest bit. How many times have you looked at a friend or colleague and thought to yourself that they're handling a bad situation much better than you would? Or maybe you see them falling to pieces over the slightest thing and write them off as being dramatic? It's almost impossible to know exactly how much stress other people are under, but you can evaluate your own levels and try to learn how to de-escalate them.

Although everyone deals with stress differently, the symptoms people suffer are often very similar. Stress can affect you physically, mentally, and emotionally in a number of different ways.

- Physical symptoms include feeling fatigued, headaches, stomach and digestive issues, difficulty sleeping, unexplained muscle aches, persistent dry mouth, loss of libido, and suffering from frequent colds or infections.
- Mental symptoms include forgetting things more easily, not being able to focus, making poor decisions, feeling anxious and worried, inability to follow a train of thought, and only seeing the negative.
- Emotional symptoms include finding it difficult to relax, being easily agitated and frustrated, having mood swings, feeling overwhelmed, having low self-esteem and feeling worthless, depression, and avoiding social situations.

You might also start behaving in a way that isn't normal for you, such as drinking more alcohol, binge eating, procrastinating and putting off tasks, biting your nails or picking your skin, and being reckless. None of these sound like a lot of fun, but it's amazing how many we can tolerate for a long time with the right coping mechanisms.

Physical Effects of Long-Term Stress

With such a huge list of stress-related symptoms, it should be easy to see how they can start to take a toll on your body. What might start as an upset stomach can eventually turn into a stomach ulcer or gastritis. Occasional heart palpitations, if left unchecked, could cause heart disease or even a heart attack. Long-term stress can also affect your skin, causing breakouts of acne, eczema, or psoriasis. Unlike the other internal symptoms, this one is easy to see but not many people recognize that it's caused by stress.

Stress also slows down your metabolism, meaning you'll find it easier to gain weight and harder to lose it. When you go into "fight-or-flight" mode, your body directs blood flow away from non-essential systems and switches them into sleep mode, like your laptop when you walk away for too long. Your digestive system is one of these because there's no need to digest food while you're in battle or running away. You might lose your appetite, find yourself craving only sugary foods, or only be able to eat smaller meals than normal while snacking in between.

Another system that stress can mess with is your reproductive system—unsurprisingly, you don't need to use this while fighting or fleeing either! In women, this can mean your menstrual cycle becomes irregular and it's also more difficult to conceive. In men, stress makes it difficult to get or keep an erection. Stress also means you're less likely to feel sexual desire and this can lead to arguments within your relationship, causing even more stress in your life.

If you start to add some of these symptoms together, you can see how long-term stress can be a killer. Combine heart disease with increased weight and you've got a recipe for disaster. Many of these issues are internal, so they might not be immediately obvious unless you pick up on the signs your body is sending you. However, feeling tired, out of breath, and having stomach aches might not immediately make you think of stress.

Learning to Spot the Signs

Your body only has so many ways to warn you that something is wrong. Pain or swelling is usually a good indicator that there's a problem and it'll tell you where that problem is, but not what's causing it. So, how do you know whether a stomach ache is caused by bad food, feeling stressed, anxiety, an ulcer, bacteria, or an inflamed appendix? That's quite the list of possible causes and some will get better on their own while others will need treatment.

Lots of illnesses and conditions have the same symptoms, for example, feeling fatigued. It's normal to be worn out when your body is fighting off a cold but if the tiredness persists for more than a few days, it might be a sign of something more serious, like anemia or low blood pressure.

Rather than looking at symptoms on their own, you need to think about what they mean together. If you didn't eat anything unusual in the last few hours, it's probably not food poisoning. Do you also have a raised temperature? If so, it might be that you've picked up a stomach bug. If you've also got a headache, you feel tired, and your mouth keeps drying up, it's probably stress.

Performing a Body Scan

You might not even notice these other symptoms unless you go looking for them. This is why it's good to get into the habit of finding a quiet moment to scan your body and see if it's trying to tell you anything. Find yourself somewhere away from other distractions and sit upright in a chair or lie flat on the bed. You want to make sure your body is in a neutral position to give you the best chance to spot any new aches and pains. Close your eyes and focus your attention on your toes. Notice how they're feeling: is there any stiffness, swelling, or pain? Flex them and make sure that they all move freely. Now move your attention to your feet and ankles, repeating the process until you reach the top of your head.

Did you notice some areas that didn't feel right? This method can help you identify muscle and joint problems, patches of dry or itchy skin, and any aches and pains. If you do it regularly, you can also pinpoint when new symptoms started. A stiff neck and a headache that appeared at the same time might be connected and due to a muscle injury, but if they started a week apart, they could be a sign of continued stress.

Eating for Health

One of the most important parts of your body to listen to is your gut. According to Ayurvedic theories, your gut is the center of your sense of purpose and direction—which is where the phrase "trust your gut" comes from. It leads you on your path and gives you the courage to make the right decision when you come to a crossroads. It's where you feel nervous (butterflies in your stomach) or excited (when your adrenaline is flowing) and it's also one of the first places to send out signals that something is wrong.

On a purely physical level, your gut is also important because it's where the process of turning food into energy begins. It's also vulnerable because it's one of the easiest places in your body for outside bacteria to access because anything you eat that is contaminated goes pretty much straight to your stomach. Outside bacteria are usually bad, however, your gut has its own healthy bacteria that work to defend against bad bacteria, help you digest your food properly, and keep the parts of your digestive system in good working order.

If you don't have a varied and healthy set of gut bacteria, you can be more vulnerable to digestive issues and outside infections. Unfortunately, many of the things we see as positive in modern life are actually not good for our gut. Keeping your house spotlessly clean, always washing your hands before eating, and spending less time outdoors means that we have fewer opportunities to pick up good bacteria from other people in our lives or from nature itself. This means many of us only have the gut bacteria we were born with so it's important to keep it healthy.

Your gut bacteria need to eat to survive but they don't get to choose their diet, that's up to you. If you eat a lot of fruit and vegetables, fiber, and probiotic foods like yogurts and some soft cheeses, your gut bacteria will be happy and healthy. However, processed foods and those with a high fat or sugar content don't contain enough nutrition for your gut bacteria and they'll die out. This means you won't digest your food as well and you'll be more prone to stomach issues.

Signs that your gut bacteria are out of balance include:

- always feeling tired
- suffering from constipation, gas, bloating, or stomach cramps
- heartburn or acid reflux
- developing a new food allergy or intolerance
- gaining or losing weight without trying
- feeling anxious, depressed, or struggling with mood swings

If any of these sound like you, it might be a sign that you need to give your gut some love and attention. Switch your diet to something that contains more whole vegetables and fruit, make sure you're getting enough sleep, and up your daily water intake. You can also take probiotic and prebiotic supplements to increase the number of healthy bacteria in your gut. Make sure you choose a good quality supplement so that you're getting the maximum benefits.

You can also help to soothe any stomach issues by taking herbal supplements or drinking soothing teas, like chamomile and ginger. Over the next few chapters you're going to find out about different herbal and homeopathic treatments and how they can help keep you healthy.

3. Nature's Pharmacy: Herbal Medicine and Essential Oils

Once upon a time, every household had its own medicine cabinet stuffed full of tinctures, ointments, salves, and teas, all made from local herbs. It was common knowledge which plants to stock to help you sleep, soothe irritated skin, or ease digestive cramps. With the arrival of mass produced pharmaceuticals, we lost this knowledge or began to treat it with suspicion. However, a renewed global interest in holistic and herbal treatments is now bringing these treatments, some of them thousands of years old, back into public knowledge. Apothecaries and herbalist shops are once again setting up shop in the high streets and there are hundreds more selling their products online.

Most herbal medicines are available in a number of forms, including capsules, dried herbs, tinctures, and teas. As mentioned in the introduction, herbal medicines are not subject to FDA approval, but the industry is self-regulating, and you'll find that most supplements suggest the same daily recommended dose. They should also list warnings on the label, as there are some herbs that should not be taken by everyone.

Growing, Foraging, and Harvesting Your Herbs

If you really want to embrace herbal medicine the old-fashioned way, there's nothing more satisfying than growing your own! It doesn't matter whether you have a lot of outside space or only a windowsill, many of the staple herbs are easy to grow and low maintenance. It can give you a real piece of mind to know exactly where your herbs have come from and that no harsh chemicals were used on them.

Setting Up Your Herb Garden

Always check the particular needs of each herb you plan to grow to make sure you can provide them with everything they need to thrive. For example, an aloe vera plant needs fairly dry, peat-free compost and lots of sun, whereas peppermint prefers to grow in moist, shady spots. If your herbs aren't native to your country, they might not survive outside and will need to be grown indoors or in a greenhouse. A good example is Bacopa or Brahmi, a small plant from India that needs to be grown in a humid environment and would struggle to grow outside in most areas of the Northern Hemisphere.

Most herbs are best sown in propagators until they are big enough to be planted outside. These are small, plastic trays with a clear lid that keeps the seeds warm and protects fragile roots from drying out. Fill your propagator with a layer of fresh compost and sprinkle your seeds evenly over the surface. Cover with a light dusting of compost and water, and leave somewhere sunny. Most plants will show signs of growth within 1-2 weeks.

Planting Out

When your herbs are a couple of inches tall and their stems are strong enough to support their own weight, it's time to transfer the seedlings into their own containers. You can use small plastic plant pots or repurpose clean yogurt pots and plastic trays—make sure you poke a few holes in the bottom so water doesn't get trapped and start to rot the soil.

Fill your new pots with compost, leaving a small dip in the center for your seedling. Carefully transfer the plant, complete with the existing soil around the roots, press the compost gently around the top, and give it a good watering. You usually only want one seedling per pot unless you plant straight into their final container. If your plants are eventually going to live outside, take time to acclimatize the seedlings by taking them outside during the day and either in again at night or by covering them in a cold frame or frost-proof covering.

After the seedlings have grown into sturdy and healthy plants, they are ready to be transplanted into their final home. Plant them in the ground or in a large tub, leaving plenty of space between each plant so they can grow. Keep watering regularly in order to maintain optimum conditions for your herbs.

Harvesting Your Herbs

Most herbs that are easy to grow at home use the flowers and leaves for medicinal purposes. This is great because they're the easiest parts to harvest, all you need is a pair of small scissors. You should harvest flowers while they're still at their best, don't wait for them to shrivel and fall off on their own, as these flowers will have fewer beneficial chemicals in them. If you're harvesting leaves, never trim them all off at once, or you will kill the plant. Take new growth leaves from the top of the stem (this means new leaves will grow in their place) and never take more than one-third at a time.

You can use both fresh and dried herbs in recipes but dried herbs last longer and are therefore easier to store. The traditional way to dry your herbs is to tie them in bunches and hang them upside down somewhere warm until all the moisture has evaporated. This can take up to two weeks for some herbs. If you're feeling impatient, you can dry them in your oven (low temperature for 30 minutes) or microwave (30-second bursts, checking in between to see if they're dry yet).

Good Herbs to Start Your Garden

Some of the easiest herbs to start growing at home are those that you use for cooking and in herbal medicine. Peppermint, cilantro, rosemary, and thyme all have nutritional and medicinal benefits and will thrive just as well in a pot on your windowsill or planted in the garden. If you want to add some color to your herb garden, look no further than lavender, chamomile, and calendula. These herbs bloom brightly and you can harvest their flowers, leaves, and stalks and use them for your own home remedies.

Wild Foraging

If you live near a natural space, you might be able to find some herbs growing in the wild. This can be an especially good way of getting hold of herbs from plants that are much larger than you'd like to grow, such as hawthorn, beech, and cedar trees. You can forage fresh leaves, berries, nuts, and fruit, but don't take any bark or roots. If you don't know how to do it safely, you could end up killing the tree, so it's best to leave a collection of these parts to the professionals.

Common Preparations

Whether you have dried your own herbs or bought them in a packet, you'll need to prepare them. This involves extracting the medicinal chemicals from the herbs and turning them into a liquid that you can easily measure and drink, much like cough syrup from the store. All you'll need are some simple pieces of equipment:put them

- sterilized glass jars
- cheesecloth or muslin for filtering
- tea strainer
- Kettle

The four different preparations covered in this chapter are infusions, decoctions, syrups, and tinctures. The first three are water based but tinctures use alcohol instead. You can also use oil as a base to make ointments and infused oils but these are only to be used externally, never eaten.

How to Make an Infusion

Infusions allow the herbs to steep in water, which extracts important vitamins and oils. You can make hot infusions—just like brewing a cup of loose-leaf tea—or cold infusions, and each method works best for different herbs. If you're using mainly flowers and leaves or moist roots, like red clover, ginger root, and raspberry leaf, use a hot infusion. A cold infusion is best for plants that already hold a lot of moisture, for example, marshmallow root, lemon balm, and rose buds.

To make a hot infusion:

1. Place three teaspoons of your chosen herbs in a tea strainer and put them in your mug.
2. Pour hot water over the herbs and cover the mug to keep in the steam.
3. Leave to steep for up to an hour—the exact time needed will depend on the herbs used—and reheat before drinking if necessary.

To make a cold infusion:

1. You'll need a 32 oz. glass jar. Fill it with cold water.
2. Add 1 oz. of herbs and stir into the water.
3. Pop the lid on tight and leave overnight.
4. Strain the mixture through the cheesecloth or muslin into another quart jar. This should remove all the herbs from the infusion.

You can store your infusions in a sealed container in the refrigerator for up to seven days. Reheat your hot infusion before drinking. Hot infusions are warming and soothing, especially if you have a cold or a sore throat. Cold infusions are refreshing, revitalizing, and delicious on hot days.

How to Make a Decoction

The differences between a decoction and a hot infusion are subtle but important. A much lower temperature is used in order to draw the goodness out of harder herbs, including bark, dried berries, seeds, and hard roots.

1. Add three teaspoons of your chosen dried herb to your saucepan and top up with 32 oz. of cold water.
2. Place your saucepan on the stove and gently heat until it is simmering nicely.
3. Cover the pan and leave for up to 45 minutes, depending on the herbs and how strong you want your decoction to be.
4. Strain the decoction into a 32 oz. glass jar but don't throw away the herbs.
5. Top up your jar by pouring more hot water through the herbs in your filter cloth.
6. If you want a sweeter flavor to your decoction, add a little raw honey, natural stevia sweetener, or fruit juice.

Decoctions can be stored in sterile jars in your refrigerator for up to a week.

How to Make a Syrup

A herbal syrup is thicker and sweeter than infusions and decoctions, which makes it particularly soothing and comforting if you have a cough or a sore throat. It also has a relatively long shelf life so you can make a large batch and keep it in the refrigerator for 3 months. All syrups use a strong decoction as a base, so you'll need to make one of those first. Then you'll add either honey or sugar to sweeten, thicken, and preserve it. Start with a 1:1 ratio of decoction and sweetener and reduce the amount of sugar or honey if you find it too sweet.

1. Return your decoction to the pan and add your choice of honey or sugar.
2. If you chose honey, gently heat the mixture until the honey dissolves but make sure it doesn't boil or this will kill the enzymes in the honey.

3. If you choose sugar, bring the mixture to a boil and simmer for 30 minutes, stirring occasionally to ensure the sugar dissolves.

4. You can now add any tinctures you have made, or add brandy at a ratio of 1 cup to every four cups of syrup. Stir it through the mixture. This step is optional but adding alcohol will make your syrup last longer.

5. Pour your syrup into sterilized glass jars, seal and place in the refrigerator to store. It's a good idea to label your syrups with the date they were made so you know how long you have to use them.

Take a spoonful of syrup to treat an illness, or add it to hot water to make a soothing hot drink. Add two spoonfuls of syrup to lemonade or soda water for a refreshing summer beverage. You can also drizzle it over ice cream, stir it into yogurt, or bake it into biscuits.

How to Make a Tincture

Tinctures have a number of advantages over water-based preparations that make them the best way to prepare your herbs. Most have a really long shelf life—they can still be good after ten years—and don't lose potency over time. Alcohol is more effective than water at extracting the plant constituents so you get a stronger medicine at the end. Different herbs need different concentrations of alcohol so make sure you always use the right combination. For tinctures using fresh herbs you need at least 75% alcohol, for dried herbs use 40-75% alcohol. The best alcohol to use is vodka but you can use brandy or anything else made from grains. Avoid anything that is flavored or colored as it won't be as pure.

To make a tincture from fresh herbs:

1. Chop your fresh herbs as small as possible and fill a glass jar with as much as you can.
2. Add your alcohol and seal the jar.
3. 24 hours later, open your jar and refill it to the top with alcohol.
4. Store your jar in a dark place for at least a month—tinctures aren't quick to make!
5. You need to strain out the herbs so pour your mixture through a fine mesh like cheesecloth to catch them. Give the material a good squeeze to get all of the liquid out of the herbs.
6. Your tincture is now ready to use.

This fresh herb tincture method works well for most leafy green herbs, for example, peppermint, oregano, lemon balm, and valerian.

To make a tincture from dry herbs:

1. Whizz your dried herbs in a blender until they resemble a fine powder.
2. Weight out 1 oz. of herbs for every 5 oz. of alcohol (remember to use lower-proof alcohol for dry herb tinctures) and mix them together in a sterilized glass jar.
3. Screw on the lid and give your jar a good shake. In fact, you'll need to shake it twice a day for the next month.
4. After a month, strain your tincture through a coffee filter to remove the herbs. If you don't use a fine strainer you'll end up with bits of herbs left in the liquid. This doesn't affect how well it works but it might taste a little grainy.

5. Bottle up your tincture and keep it in your cupboard for when it's needed.

Dry herb tinctures work really well for aromatic herbs, like lavender, or herbs that you usually buy already dried or powdered, like cardamom and cinnamon.

Tinctures don't taste anywhere near as nice as infusions and teas but they work faster because alcohol is absorbed straight into the bloodstream rather than making its way through your digestive system. To avoid the strong alcohol burning your mouth, dilute a few drops of tincture in a tablespoon of water.

The Essentials on Oils

Another popular way to harness the healing power of nature is through essential oils. These are extremely concentrated plant extracts and it takes a huge amount of herb to produce enough oil to fill a small jar. They're difficult to make at home, not only because of the quantity of herb needed but also because you'd need expensive distillation equipment. However, they're readily available online, in healthcare shops, and in herbal apothecaries.

Unlike the other herbal preparations detailed above, you don't ingest essential oils. You can massage or diffuse them into your skin and breathe in their scent. Lots of oils are available as small roll-ons that you can rub into pulse points like your wrists and temples. Because they're so potent you only need to use a small amount at a time to feel the benefit.

Essential oils are available in pure form or as diluted solutions. If you want to apply the oils to your skin, you must use a diluted version, or they could cause skin irritation. You can do this yourself by mixing a few drops with a carrier oil, such as jojoba, almond, or coconut oil. Essential oils that are sold as roll-ons, massage oils, or body sprays are already diluted and, therefore, safe to use.

Top Five Oils to Make You Feel Good

If you're wondering which oils to start your collection with, these options are reasonably inexpensive, easy to find, and have lots of benefits.

Lavender Oil

This is a gentle oil that is tolerated by most people, including children and infants. Lavender oil is well-known as a sleep aid and can be added to your evening bath to help you relax and unwind. It's often sold as a pillow spray or a roll-on for your temple.

Peppermint

Peppermint oil can reduce headaches, improve your mood, and help you feel less tired. When rubbed into skin it's also an effective cleaner, removing bacteria and treating fungal infections like athlete's foot.

Rosemary

Rosemary oil, if rubbed into your joints, can help to reduce inflammation and pain. It's also great for reducing stress and helping you feel more positive, as well as improving brain function. However, if you're pregnant, suffer from high blood pressure, or have epilepsy, rosemary oil can have some negative effects so it's best avoided.

Cedarwood

Add a few drops of diluted cedarwood oil to your shampoo or shower gel to leave your hair and skin looking and smelling great.

It's a great natural treatment for anxiety and sleep issues like insomnia. Pop a few drops in a diffuser by your bed to help you drift off at the end of a long day.

Eucalyptus

This essential oil is a particularly effective treatment for colds and blocked noses. Add a few drops to hot water and breathe in the steam for almost instant relief. It's also a wonderful treatment for cold sores if you rub a small amount of diluted oil onto the affected area.

Unlike herbal medicines, it's not recommended to use essential oils on a regular basis. This is because your body can get used to them and they will become less effective. Instead, use them as part of an indulgent treat; pop a little oil in the bath or in your diffuser while you relax and you'll find your mind and spirits instantly lifted.

4. Nature's Pharmacy: Treatments for Common Ailments

R ecipes for herbal treatments have been passed on by word of mouth for thousands of years. The Ancient Greeks, Egyptians, and Chinese all started cataloging and writing them down, but it was a painstaking process as each copy had to be made by hand. With the invention of the printing press, books on herbalism were easier to find, and it was pretty unusual for a household not to have one. The renewed interest in herbalist literature means people can once again have instant access to generations' worth of gentle and effective medicines.

Instead of filling your cupboards with pharmaceutical tablets, creams, and syrups, stock them with some of the following herbs so you'll always have something on hand for any emergency.

Pain and Inflammation

Almost everyone takes painkillers. They're a universal treatment for everything from headaches to a sprained ankle. The first commercial painkiller, aspirin, is still made from the chemicals found naturally in willow bark, which had been used for thousands of years as an herbal remedy. You can buy willow bark today and chew it for quick pain relief, or try one of these other healing herbs.

Turmeric

This medicinal herb has its roots in Ayurveda medicine and TCM. It is extracted from the rhizome of the plant and is a rich source of a chemical called curcumin, which is known to have strong anti-inflammatory and antioxidant powers. It works to reduce inflammation by blocking signals that tell your tissues to swell up. This also lessens the pain you feel in your joints as less inflamed tissue means they can move more easily.

Turmeric is one of the easiest herbs to find in the shops because it's also used as a powdered spice to flavor food. You can use the same powder to make a warm, soothing turmeric latte—stir 1 tsp of turmeric powder into 1 1/2 cups of warm milk and enjoy. You can also buy turmeric as a fresh root, much like its close relation to ginger, and you can grate it, chop it up, or blend it into a paste for use in recipes.

As well as reducing joint inflammation, turmeric is also very effective at treating digestive discomfort by calming any inflammation and irritation in the lining of your stomach and intestines. It also helps promote healthy gut bacteria because it's prebiotic. Scientists and herbalists agree that it's better to ingest turmeric by adding it to your cooking rather than taking supplements where the concentration of turmeric is unnecessarily high (Brown, 2022). Turmeric has been known to increase your risk of developing kidney stones, and it also reduces the effectiveness of some painkillers and chemotherapy drugs.

Cloves

Clove oil is a traditional remedy to help with toothache and can be safely rubbed onto the affected area. It's so safe you can even use it on children and pets. You might even find it added to commercial mouthwash, partly for its medicinal use and also because it tastes good! This is another herb that you can add to your cooking to boost not only the flavor of your dishes but also your well-being.

You can buy clove as the aforementioned oil or as dried buds (most usually for cooking), but the flowers and stems can also be used. If you grow your own cloves, this means you can use the whole flowering plant so that you won't have a lot of wastage. Cloves come from the clove tree, a tropical plant native to Indonesia, and will grow well in warm, humid conditions.

The active ingredient in clove oil is called eugenol and it works in the same way as turmeric: by blocking the messages in your body that tell your tissues to become inflamed. Cloves can also lower your blood sugar levels, so don't take it if you are also taking medication for diabetes without discussing it with your doctor first. Adding more clove to your diet as part of a nutritional plan to control diabetes or pre-diabetes may be beneficial if monitored correctly.

Valerian

This herb is native to Europe and Asia, but thanks to past travelers taking it with them, it was transported all over the world and now grows nearly everywhere. The medicinal part of the plant is the root, which is harvested after at least two years of growth. Scientists are still investigating exactly how valerian root works, but they think it includes compounds that increase brain chemicals like gamma-aminobutyric acid (GABA), which make you feel calm.

Valerian is a versatile herb and could be listed under several different categories. One of its main benefits is as a sedative, and it helps fight pain by making tense muscles relax. It specifically targets tension headaches caused when head and neck muscles contract, and it's also useful for fighting menstrual cramps and inflammation.

It is also hugely beneficial for treating mental health conditions like anxiety, insomnia, and stress. However, if you're already taking pharmaceutical drugs for these conditions, you shouldn't take valerian root as well. It can increase the effects of these medications and make you feel more drowsy and depressed.

Rosemary

Rosemary is a favorite herb for flavoring dishes from the Mediterranean region of Europe and it's also easy to grow at home, either as a windowsill plant or part of an outside herb garden. It smells fantastic and attracts bees, which then help to pollinate the rest of your garden. You can harvest the thin needle leaves and either dry them or use them fresh.

This herb has pain-relieving and anti-inflammatory properties and is most effective as an essential oil that can be rubbed into sore muscles or swollen joints. Rosemary oil can also help you feel less stressed, which means it's doubly great at relieving tension headaches and chronic pain. Rosemary can also have a beneficial effect on your brain as it's been shown to help prevent brain aging and protect against brain damage, especially in patients who have suffered a stroke (Seyedemadi et al., 2016).

If you're just adding it to your food, it's going to be difficult to ingest enough rosemary to cause any negative side effects, so it's an extremely safe herb to use. Before taking any supplements in capsule form, check with your doctor if you are on blood thinners or diuretics, as rosemary can interfere with them.

Cayenne

You might recognize this herb as a type of pepper that gives chili its distinctive fiery taste, but it's also one of the most useful herbs for reducing pain from inflammation. This is because the chemical capsaicin—the one that makes your tongue tingle—has wonderful anti-inflammatory properties. You can find it in many commercial creams, but it's also really easy to make your own at home; just follow the recipe below.

Capsaicin blocks the nerves in the affected area from sending signals to the brain that you're in pain. It also warms your skin when you rub it in, which can be soothing. There is a slight risk that if you use the cream too much, you'll get used to it, and it won't be as effective as it was. If this happens, try something else for a couple of weeks and then return to the cream, but use it less frequently.

Capsaicin Cream

- 1 cup of coconut oil
- 1/2 cup of olive oil
- 3 tbsp of cayenne powder
- heatproof glass bowl
- coffee filter paper
- sterilized glass jar for storage

Put the olive oil and the cayenne pepper in the heatproof glass bowl and suspend it over a saucepan of boiling water. Stir the mixture and simmer for 15 minutes at a medium heat. This creates a hot infusion of capsaicin in oil. Remove the bowl and let it cool for half an hour, and then strain it into the glass jar using the filter paper. Microwave the coconut oil for 20 seconds and stir it into the oil infusion. Pop it into the refrigerator and leave it to set for at least half an hour. Keep it in the refrigerator and check for signs of spoiling. Your cream should be kept for at least a couple of months, but discard if discoloration or separation occurs, or you notice it smells off.

Digestive Health

Getting hold of good-quality food today is expensive, but the cheaper, processed options are playing havoc with our digestive systems. The number of food allergies seems to be on the rise (Jones, 2020), indicating that something in our digestive systems is changing for the worse. When irritation strikes, these herbs will help calm down inflammation and restore balance to your gut.

Ginger

This useful herb originally came from China but is now also farmed in India and parts of Africa. The part used in herbal medicine is the rhizome. This is a sort of underground stem that the roots grow from and can be harvested without causing damage to the plant. You can buy fresh ginger from your local grocery store: fresh root in the grocery section and in powdered form among the jars of herbs and spices.

According to Ayurveda, ginger is a warming herb that provides heat to the stomach and allows it to digest food more effectively. This effect comes from the compound gingerol which helps to keep food moving through your stomach and intestines. Problems like bloating, gas, and nausea can occur when food sits in the stomach for too long, so if you find you're suffering after a meal, try a cup of ginger tea to pep up the digestive process.

Ginger can be added to your cooking or taken as a supplement. Ginger biscuits have long been recommended to help relieve the symptoms of morning sickness during pregnancy, and ginger cake or carrot and ginger soup are also delicious ways to boost your digestive health.

Gentian

A tall, yellow plant from the mountainous regions of Europe, Gentian has been curing stomach complaints for thousands of years. It's part of a group of herbs known as bitter herbs because of their distinctive bitter taste. Bitter herbs make great digestive tonics because they stimulate the production of digestive fluids, including saliva, bile, and hydrochloric acid.

Gentian also has a beneficial effect on your liver and can help it function at its best. By stimulating bile production it helps to clear waste products from your liver and increases your body's ability to break down and digest fats and fatty acids.

One problem with bitter herbs is that they are unpleasant to take. You can counter their bitter taste by combining them with other, more pleasantly flavored herbs or adding sugar or natural honey to teas and infusions. You can buy gentian from specialist herbalists as a dried powder or a ready-made tincture.

Chamomile

One of the gentlest herbs there is, chamomile, which is even safe to be used by young babies, but that doesn't mean it is less effective than the others on this list. In fact, it's been the first herb people turn to for calming digestive discomfort for thousands of years. A small, white daisy-like flower on feathery leaves, chamomile is easy to grow and harvest at home and should be a staple of every herb garden. Found growing naturally in Eastern Europe and Western Asia, chamomile has a long history in both Western and Eastern herbalist traditions.

Chamomile is a cooling herb with anti-inflammatory and anti-spasmodic properties. Rather than stimulating digestion, it works by calming inflammation and halting stomach spasms caused by contracting muscles. It is an effective and natural way to deal with the symptoms of colic in infants. In adults, use chamomile to soothe peptic ulcers, gastritis, and any other inflammation or irritation.

You can use chamomile flowers in a salad where their sweet flavor provides a lovely contrast to peppery arugula. Another popular way to ingest chamomile is as a tea infusion. You can buy chamomile tea bags or dried herbs to make your own.

Fennel

Another gentle, cooling herb, fennel, comes from Europe and Asia but is easy to grow anywhere. Its green leaves resemble the fluffy tops of a wild carrot, and it has a lovely flavor that makes it a popular ingredient for cooks all over the world. You can eat the leaves, seeds, and bulbs that grow underneath the ground, and both have medicinal properties.

Fennel is widely recognized as one of the oldest medicinal herbs (Lubeck, 2023). It is antispasmodic and anti-inflammatory and can be used to effectively reduce the symptoms of bloating, cramping, and irritable bowel syndrome. It can also help to disperse trapped gas, and its antimicrobial properties mean it helps to look after the good bacteria in your gut. Because it helps to calm muscle spasms, fennel has also been shown to have a beneficial effect on menstrual cramps.

You can buy dried fennel to mix into a drink for infants to help relieve digestive discomfort, help them pass gas, and keep bowel movements regular. You can usually find fresh fennel in the grocery store along with dried fennel seeds and fennel spice. This is a great herb to mix with bitter herbs, like gentian, to mask their taste.

Marshmallow Root

This delicate flowering herb is native to the wetlands and marshes of Europe and Asia. Like the areas where it grows, it has a cooling and wet energy, which is perfect for looking after the soft tissues of your digestive system from your mouth to your gut. These tissues are more fragile than the skin on the outside of your body and, therefore, more easily damaged. Marshmallow root can help to keep these tissues moist and lined in a healthy mucus.

Marshmallow root is also an effective treatment for conditions that come from having an excess of stomach acid like gastritis and heartburn. It repairs the mucus layer between the inflamed skin in your throat and stomach and the stomach acid which makes it sore. With this added protection your digestive tract can have time to heal without being burned. It works in the same way to help relieve the discomfort of a sore throat, and the next time you have one, you can try this homemade tea blend, which is equally comforting and soothing.

Marshmallow and Cinnamon Tea

- 60g of dried marshmallow root
- 25g of cinnamon powder
- 15g of dried citrus peel
- 10 whole cloves
- 10 cups of water
- Coffee filter paper

This recipe makes enough for three or four cups of tea which can be reheated over the course of the day. Discard any remaining tea after 36 hours.Put all the dried ingredients in a saucepan and bring to a boil. Reduce the heat and simmer for 30-40 minutes. Pour the tea through the filter paper to remove the herbs. If you want to make it a little sweeter, stir a teaspoon of honey into each cup.

Mental Health and Better Sleep

We all wish we could get more sleep. Whether it's the kids, work, or worries keeping you awake, it makes navigating the days so much harder if you're always feeling tired. It's often not as easy as just going to bed early, and this can sometimes be down to issues without mental health. A huge part of holistic medicine deals with helping people to unwind, let go of problems, and learn to value their own needs. Getting away from the noise of modern life is difficult, but these herbs can help.

Passionflower

There are more than 500 varieties of passion flowers, all instantly recognizable by their distinctive flowers with protruding stamen in the shape of a cross. It is these flowers that are dried to make the medicinal herb. This climbing vine is native to the southern

United States, central, and south America but was transported to Europe by Spanish settlers in the 17th century. It was used in Western European herbal medicine as a sedative and sleep aid, and today, it persists as a treatment for mild anxiety.

Passionflower is thought to work by helping to increase the levels of GABA in your brain. Higher levels of GABA help lower the activity levels of your brain—a bit like closing some of the open tabs in your internet browser—and this makes it easier for you to fall asleep because there is less "noise" in your brain. This is also how it lowers anxiety levels. Because passionflower is a milk sedative it can sometimes make you feel sleepy or drowsy, so don't take it alongside other sedatives, sleeping tablets, or anti-anxiety medication.

You can buy passionflower as a liquid extract or dried flowers, which make a delicious, sweet tea. Drink it before bedtime to help your brain switch off at the end of a busy day.

Ashwagandha

One of the most important herbs in Ayurvedic practice, ashwagandha has been used for thousands of years. It is a versatile tonic that boosts your overall mental and physical health. It also treats a number of different conditions, including anxiety, high blood pressure, and arthritic swelling. The parts of the plant that are used for medicinal purposes are the root and dried seeds. It's difficult to grow this shrub outside of the warm Indian climate but capsules, gummies, and powdered herbs are easy to buy online or from your local herbalist store.

Because ashwagandha is such a well-used herb there have been many scientific studies conducted to see if it really works to reduce levels of anxiety and stress.. According to the research

(Office of Dietary Supplements - Ashwagandha: Is It Helpful for Stress, Anxiety, or Sleep? 2023), the answer is a resounding yes! These studies have also shown that ashwagandha seems to have a soothing effect on the brain, similar to passionflower, which can help you fall asleep more easily.

Ashwagandha may have an adverse effect if taken with other anti-anxiety drugs so always talk to your healthcare provider before taking a new supplement. The powder mixes easily into warmed milk for a soothing bedtime drink and you can add a little honey, vanilla essence, or natural stevia sweetener to mask the slightly bitter taste.

St John's

This herb is native to Europe and grows into a small shrub with bright yellow flowers that are collected, along with the leaves, and used for herbal supplements. It's most commonly available as a tincture or as a tablet. St John's wort can be as effective at treating anxiety and depression as prescription medication like Prozac and Zoloft. It increases the amount of a hormone called serotonin, which is read by your brain and can make you feel calm and happy. The effect comes from two compounds found in the plant called hypericin and hyperforin.

St John's wort is very well researched but it also interacts negatively with some common pharmaceuticals, so be careful with this one if you are taking oral contraceptives, antidepressants, prescription painkillers, or are on a prescribed course of other drugs. Always speak to your doctor before taking St John's wort as it might not be suitable for you. Do not stop taking St John's wort suddenly, even if you experience side effects you don't like, as you can suffer withdrawal symptoms.

Lavender

You might already associate lavender with a good night's sleep because this is one of the most well-known herbal remedies. You can buy baby wash, pillow sprays, and pulse point roll-ons, all made with lavender essential oils and designed to help you fall asleep. Lavender oil works best when absorbed directly into the skin so rub some diluted essential oil into your wrists, collar bones, or temples before going to bed. Unlike other sleep-enhancing medications, lavender doesn't have any side effects, and it won't leave you feeling drowsy the following day.

As well as being an effective sleep aid, lavender has a wonderful, distinctive smell that is relaxing to breathe in from the live plant as well as from the essential oil. Lavender comes from the Mediterranean region of Europe and Africa but it's hardy and will grow in most gardens. You can harvest the small purple flowers and dry them at home to create potpourri or put them into little bags and pop them in your drawers to keep your clothes freshly scented.

Scientists believe that lavender works by increasing how much GABA your brain absorbs. This makes you feel calm and relaxed and slows down your brain so you can get to sleep without being disturbed by excess thoughts.

Sage

Another common herb that's easy to grow in your garden or on a windowsill, sage is full of vitamins, minerals, and nutrients. It's also rich in antioxidants and can lower your cholesterol levels if taken regularly. Adding sage to your food or drinking sage tea is the easiest way to get all of the goodness from this Mediterranean herb. If you grow your own, you can dry the herbs at home and add them to soups, sauces, and stews.

Sage is a wonderful tonic for brain health and can help to stop brain aging and memory loss. Scientists have tested how sage extract can help patients with mild Alzheimer's, and the results show that their memory and brain function actually improved (Akhondzadeh et al., 2003). They think that it stops important brain chemicals from breaking down, keeping it healthier for longer.

Because sage works best when taken every day—unlike other herbs that are used to treat illnesses or calm acute situations—you should try and find ways to incorporate it into your cooking. Try this easy sage honey recipe to add a brain boost to your breakfast.

Sage Honey

- Raw honey
- Dried sage leaves
- Sterilized glass jar
- Fine mesh strainer

Place the whole dried sage leaves in the bottom of the jar until it is roughly 1/3 full. Pour over the honey and stir so everything is mixed well. Top up with more honey if needed and seal the jar securely. Cover the jar and leave the honey to sit for at least five days, occasionally turning it upside down to ensure an even mix between the honey and the leaves. After five days, taste the mixture and either leave it for a bit longer (if you want a stronger sage flavor) or strain out the herbs and discard. Your honey will keep for a very long time so you can reap the benefits of your sage infusion for months.

Herbal Tonics

As a society, we are used to reactionary medicine: you get a headache, so you take some painkillers, or you cut your hand and apply a band-aid. However, a lot of herbal medicines are tonics, small amounts that you take every day to maintain your health and improve your well-being. If you take vitamin supplements or take a walk every day, these are holistic tonics that don't treat a specific symptom or condition but instead work to prevent illnesses from occurring.

Herbal tonics are designed to be gentle and support your body's functions. It's like keeping the oil in your car topped up or replacing batteries in your remote before they run out. It can be difficult to know if an herbal tonic is working because you won't see a sudden and beneficial change. Instead, you'll need to check in with your body over time, and you should soon see that you're picking up fewer colds, suffering from fever aches and pains, and less prone to conditions like high blood pressure, high cholesterol, and anxiety.

Schisandra

Schisandra is almost idolized in TCM for its ability to treat every part of the body. It appears in all the ancient texts and has been helping to keep people in top condition for thousands of years. The plant is a large vine with small red berries, and it's these berries that form the medicinal herb. Schisandra's Chinese name means "five-flavor berries and these flavors refer to the key elements of TCM—salty, sweet, bitter, pungent, and sour—and Schisandra is the only herb in TCM, so they contain them. Practitioners believe it is this quality that allows the herb to be a universal tonic.

One of Schisandra's best qualities is that it's what's known as an adaptogen. These herbs help to restore balance, especially after times of stress, by raising or lowering levels of chemicals in the body as needed. Prolonged feelings of stress can upset many bodily functions, so taking adaptogenic herbs is vital to preserve normal activity.

As well as aiding with stress relief, Schisandra also benefits the liver, brain, immune system, and skin. It is rich in antioxidants which can help support your body as you get older and reduce some of the effects of aging. Schisandra is readily available as a tincture and can be added to drinks or taken neat as a daily tonic over an extended period of time.

Dandelion

Most people want to remove the dandelions from their gardens, but this resilient weed is actually one of the best herbal tonics, and it improves almost every part of your life. Dandelions are found all over the world and they're harvested for their roots, leaves, and flowers, all of which act on different parts of the body. The roots boost your liver function and make sure that it keeps disposing of bodily waste efficiently. The leaves have a similarly stimulating effect on your kidneys and are a natural diuretic. The flowers can help to lift your mood, especially in the dark and cold winter months.

Dandelion leaves and flowers can be eaten fresh and are great in a healthy salad. Alternatively, you can harvest and dry them from your garden and brew them in a delicious and revitalizing dandelion tea. The root has a bitter flavor and is best combined in a tincture or decoction with other tonic herbs to mask its taste. If you mix several herbs together, try and choose those that act on the body in the same way: this will amplify the result.

Dandelion Flower Iced Tea

- A quart of fresh dandelion flowers
- Paper towels
- Large glass bowl
- Pitcher with a lid
- Lemon juice

Rinse your dandelion flowers under running cold water and pat them dry with paper towels. Meanwhile, boil a cup of water and pour it into the large glass bowl. Add the flowers and leave them to steep for up to ten minutes. Remove the flowers, pour the tea into the pitcher, and refrigerate for at least four hours. Serve with lemon juice and ice for a refreshing and uplifting drink.

Immune Boosters

Your immune system is a collection of organs, glands, hormones, and cells that all work together to fight off infection and keep your body in good condition. Sometimes it can benefit from a little help, and that's where these helpful herbs come in.

Echinacea

This distinctive purple flower is native to North America and formed an important part of Native American Herbalism for many different tribes. Everything from the flower to the root has its uses, but where echinacea really excels is in modulating your immune system's response. It can kick start your immune response or help your system to wind down if it's still on the attack even after defeating all the invading pathogens. You can take echinacea as a preventative measure if you know you're going to be visiting someone who isn't well or if you're worried about catching a cold or the flu.

Echinacea can also help you recover faster if you do find yourself feeling under the weather. It does this by stimulating the production of white blood cells. Echinacea also has potent antimicrobial properties which make it effective at killing viruses and bacteria in your mouth and throat when you drink it or gargle with it. You'll know it's working because it will leave you with a cool, tingly feeling, much like strong mint, which can feel soothing on a sore throat. Echinacea works best when taken in liquid form like a tincture, liquid extract, or decoction, and you can add it to a drink of your choice to make it more palatable if needed.

Lemon Balm

Another popular kitchen herb that gives dishes a lemony flavor, lemon balm is also a powerful antiviral that can actually stop viruses from getting into your cells and multiplying. Found growing all over the Mediterranean region of Europe, as well as central Asia, lemon balm will be equally happy in your home herb garden. The leaves can be harvested and eaten or prepared as tea or tincture. If you opt for the tincture, you can also apply it straight to cold sores to treat them topically.

Recent studies have shown that lemon balm essential oil is extremely effective at combating a wide range of viruses, from mild colds to avian flu and even HIV-1 (Islam et al., 2022). This means it will reduce symptoms and speed up your immune system's response. Lemon balm should be your go-to herb if you're feeling run down and struggling with a succession of colds, coughs, and sore throats, especially through the damp winter months.

Lemon balm also has a calming effect on your nervous system, meaning it can be useful for reducing the symptoms of mild anxiety. It can also help with mild depressive episodes by improving your mood.

Thyme

Also from the Mediterranean region of Europe, thyme was a popular herb with the Ancient Greeks and Egyptians, both of whom used it in religious ceremonies because of its strong scent. It's also very tasty and you can find it as an ingredient in a lot of cuisine from the same area. Thyme is used a lot in food like stews and pasta sauces which are thought of as warming and comforting, and that's exactly what this herb is. Thyme helps stimulate digestion by warming the stomach and it also helps to dry out "wet" illnesses like colds and chesty coughs.

Thyme contains a high concentration of volatile oils and these have a strong antimicrobial action. Taking a liquid extract or inhaling the vapors from a hot infusion will instantly kill any microbes taking up residence in your throat or nasal passages—great if you've been around a lot of germs lately. Thyme and lemon balm grow nicely together, so keep them both in your herb garden and you'll never be bothered by viruses and bacteria again!

Lemon and Thyme Herbal Tea

- 1 tbsp. of fresh lemon balm leaves
- 1/2 tbsp. of fresh thyme leaves
- honey (optional)
- heatproof bowl
- mug or tea cup
- fine mesh strainer

Place the fresh herbs into the heatproof bowl and pour over a cup of freshly boiled water. Leave to steep for five minutes (ten minutes if you like a stronger flavor) so that the water can extract the goodness from the leaves. Pop your strainer over your favorite mug or tea cup and pour the tea through, removing the herbs and leaving you with a delicious healing brew. Add honey to sweeten it if you prefer, or enjoy it as is.

5. Alternative Treatments: Homeopathy and Flower Remedies

The scientific and medical knowledge we have today has resulted from millennia of research, experimentation, and study. Over that time, many ideas have been modified or replaced, such as the idea that the Earth is flat or at the center of the universe. In the quest for new and more effective medical treatments, doctors have repeatedly turned back to herbal and holistic therapies and combined this knowledge with current medical practices to develop new systems of treatment. Homeopathy is one of these systems.

Principles and History of Homeopathy

Popularized in the late 18th century by a German doctor named Samuel Hahnemann, homeopathy blends herbal knowledge with some of the philosophies of the Ancient Greek physician Hippocrates. Hippocrates was responsible for cataloging a lot of herbal treatments, as well as writing the first medical books to explain how the body worked and how diseases could be treated. He actually got in a lot of trouble during his lifetime for presenting his opinions—such as diseases occurring naturally, not as the result of curses or the will of the gods—even though they were later proven to be mostly correct.

One of Hippocrates' ideas was that "like cures like." What he meant is that if you're suffering from symptoms of an illness, they can be cured by taking medicine that produces the same effects. For example, if you have a fever, eating pepper—which warms you up and can make you sweat in high concentrations—can help to reduce the fever. Hahnemann took this sentiment and turned it into the first key principle of homeopathy.

In preparing his homeopathic treatments, Hahnemann took great inspiration from the vast knowledge of the herbalist community. It was already well-known that chamomile helped with colic and arnica could reduce swelling, but Hahnemann looked for a way to improve the effectiveness of these treatments and make them easy to reproduce. Homeopathy isn't just another form of plant medicine, though, it also uses minerals and metals like magnesium and zinc.

The second key principle of homeopathy is that less is more: The more a treatment is diluted, the more potent it becomes. Hahnemann reasoned that taking a minute dose of medication would kick-start the body's immune response and cause it to heal itself, rather than relying on modern medicine to calm symptoms or relieve pain. This is better because modern medicine only treats the physical aspects of an illness, but homeopathic medicines also help to stimulate your vital life force and provide healing energy, which your body utilizes in its healing journey.

Like the other medicinal practices that have already been explored, homeopathy is a holistic form of healing. When you book a consultation with a homeopath, they will ask you all about your lifestyle so they can match you to the best treatments. They'll want to know how you feel in general, what your diet is like, and the current state of your emotional well-being. They might offer counseling sessions alongside their prescribed remedies and suggest you book a series of follow-up appointments so they can judge how well the medication is working.

Why Choose Homeopathic Treatments?

Homeopathic medicines are extremely mild, and so don't produce side effects or interact badly with other prescription medications. They come in liquid form and as small pills that are easy to swallow, especially for children and the elderly. As part of the dilution process, the extractions—the first extraction, made from the original healing source and alcohol, called the mother tincture—are vigorously shaken to imprint the energy of the healing tincture onto the water itself. The more dilutions the remedy goes through, the stronger the energy imprint left behind, even if there is very little of the physical herb or mineral left. This is why the stronger (more diluted) medicines have a greater effect on healing your energy and your inner self.

A good example to use here would be the homeopathic remedy arnica. Distilled from the poisonous arnica plant, this remedy is prescribed to reduce bruising and swelling. You can buy many non-homeopathic creams containing arnica that are used topically to reduce the appearance of a bruise. Taking the homeopathic arnica pills will also work internally to heal any emotional or spiritual bruising that may also have occurred; for example, if the bruise was caused by falling from the loft ladder, you might start to feel anxious about using it again if that emotional bruise is not healed as well.

Many conditions simply don't have reliable treatments, and some people have to turn to alternative therapies for relief. Fibromyalgia and myalgic encephalomyelitis (ME) are illnesses that cause huge amounts of distress to those who suffer from them, and yet there is very little that modern medicine can do to offer relief. Homeopathy offers another option.

Homeopathy and Science

All of the holistic treatments in this book have been subjected to various scientific studies and produced a wide range of results. Some, like the abilities of rosemary to prevent brain aging or lemon balm to speed up your recovery from the flu, have been analyzed and evaluated, and scientists know exactly how and why they work. Others, like how ashwagandha makes you feel calm, are still a mystery: Scientists will agree that it does work, but they can't explain how! Then there's the group of alternative therapies that, according to our understanding of science, don't have any effects at all, even though millions of people have felt the benefits. Homeopathy, acupuncture, and osteopathy fall into this category.

If there's no scientific backing for homeopathy, why is it still so popular? It's not that practitioners are trying to deny science, but there are so many things that science hasn't been able to provide an explanation for—why we dream, why we yawn, and what consciousness is, to name but a few—that they don't believe we should discount the unexplainable. Our bodies are full of energy and electricity, and without them, we will die, so it makes sense that disruptions in their flow can cause medical problems and require medical treatments.

Many scientists explain away the testimony of people who have responded well to homeopathic treatments by saying they're just experiencing a placebo effect. However, the point of homeopathic remedies is to help the body to heal itself and a placebo effect means that your body has healed itself, so what exactly is there to complain about? At the end of the day, holistic medicine is meant to improve your life, and whether that comes from a chemical response or a placebo effect, the end result is still the same. If you find something that helps you improve your health or find peace of mind, then it works, even if no one can explain why.

Don't Discard Modern Treatments Entirely

Even the most devout followers of homeopathy will tell you that the remedies have limits. In some cases, there is no substitute for a course of treatment prescribed by your doctor, for example, most chemotherapy medications. Where homeopathy, like herbal medicines, can help aid the process by reducing side effects and keeping you mentally, emotionally, and spiritually healthy. Under no circumstances should you stop taking life-saving medication that has been prescribed for you by a licensed medical practitioner in favor of taking homeopathic remedies instead.

While some conditions, like diabetes and polycystic ovary syndrome, can be managed holistically through herbal or homeopathic medication and lifestyle changes, you should still make the switch under the guidance of your doctor and a licensed holistic practitioner. You absolutely have the right to decide on your own treatment, but no one should be making such changes without discussing it with the experts first.

Medicine Cabinet Must-Haves

Homeopathic remedies are easily available. You don't need a prescription and will find them on the shelf in most pharmacies alongside painkillers, vitamins, and creams. However, these are likely to only be the most common remedies, so if your homeopath suggests you should take something a little more unusual, you will probably need to visit a specialist homeopathic pharmacy. A quick online search should help you find one near you, but if there isn't a local option, many of them will also deliver if you place an order through their website.

Most homeopathic remedies are taken as a small sugar pill that has absorbed the mother's tincture. It is placed under the tongue and allowed to dissolve and be absorbed into the body. The strength of the remedy is denoted by a number and letter after its name, e.g., arnica 30C or gelsemium 1M. The most common options that you can buy yourself are 6C, 30C, 200C, and 1M, although stronger preparations are available on prescription from your homeopath. Make sure you follow the recommended dose as written on the bottle or directed by your homeopath so that the remedy can be most effective.

Generally, 30C remedies are used for occasional treatments and are safe for you to self-medicate. 1M remedies are for more acute treatments, as they are considered to be much stronger. In order to build your homeopathic home pharmacy, consider stocking up on 30C or 200C versions of some of the following remedies: They have an exceedingly long shelf-life, so you don't need to worry about having to throw away unused medications.

Arnica

This remedy is for trauma, both physical and emotional. Arnica encourages the body to heal from bruises, muscle aches, and injuries caused by falls, bumps, surgery, and accidents. It also helps to heal emotional bruises, like shock, and can be particularly useful for patients who try to avoid seeking help because they would rather avoid unwanted attention.

Nux Vomica

Keep this in your medical cupboard for moments of overindulgence or excess. Particularly useful at settling digestive discomforts if you've had too much to eat or drink, it can also be used to calm the stomach if it's unsettled by other medication you have to take like chemotherapy drugs or steroids to treat an autoimmune condition. Nux vomica can also help you to recover from a period of overwork and stress caused by stretching yourself too thin.

Rhus Tox

Like arnica, rhus tox is recommended for the treatment of sore muscles and joints, but with a focus on those caused by inflammation and swelling, including arthritis. It is also useful in helping the body heal from skin irritations, rashes, and conditions like chickenpox and shingles. You can take it alongside arnica for sprains and strains for an extra boost of healing power.

Chamomilla

Made from chamomile extract, this remedy is for acute and unbearable pain and the irritability that comes with it. Chamomilla is often recommended for children who suffer from colic, teething pain, or recurring earaches. It also works for adults and can help soothe menstrual cramps, labor pains, and lingering pain after surgery or dental procedures.

Ignatia

An important remedy for emotional healing, take Ignatia to help your body heal from grief, both sudden and acute, and that which you've been holding onto for a long time. Grief can be the unex-pected cause of a number of mental health worries such as anxiety, depression, insomnia, anguish, and homesickness, but a trained homeopath will be able to recommend Ignatia by finding out all about you.

Gelsemium

This should be your first port of call when you come down with a miserable case of influenza, especially one that starts to build up over the course of a few days. Gelsemium can help to reduce the effects of the fever, shakes and chills, aching muscles, headaches, and that horrible viral fatigue that makes the flu feel like it's lasting forever. It also has a secondary use for feelings of anxiety around a specific event, like an appointment at the dentist or a public speaking engagement.

Aconite

Aconite works quickly, so it should be taken at the first sign of a problem. It's excellent at prompting emotional recovery from shock and can also help bring you out of a panic attack. Aconite can also help with conditions that come on suddenly, giving your body a shock, like fevers, headaches, and sore throats.

Belladonna

A well-known poison from the foxglove plant, belladonna's healing qualities come from its ability to battle inflammation, pain, and swelling. Take it if you have a wound that becomes infected, an abscess, or any other inflammation that is accompanied by throbbing pain and heat. It's also great at bringing down fevers and helping you recover from sunstroke or sunburn.

Apis

Apis is every traveler's best friend because it provides relief from insect bites and stings. Like belladonna, apis is for red, hot swellings, but looks for a stinging pain rather than one that throbs. You can also use it for any skin conditions that come out in a rash, like urticaria and hives, or those caused by an allergic reaction. If your skin is red and itchy, turn to apis for relief.

Hepar Sulph

This remedy is versatile and covers a number of uses, making it an important ingredient in any home remedy cabinet. Firstly, Hepar sulph gives you another great option for treating infections and inflammations, especially those that produce pus, because it has antibiotic qualities. Secondly, it is very effective at stimulating your body to heal from coughs, sore throats, and other ailments of the respiratory system as such, it is one of the few homeopathic remedies specifically recommended for treating cases of croup in children.

Cantharis

Another multifunctional remedy, cantharis is best used to treat burning and stinging pain, whatever the cause. Skin burns and blisters, including those caused by sunburn, can be soothed by cantharis ointment or by taking this remedy in pill form. It's also a wonderful treatment for cystitis, especially if drinking cold drinks makes you feel worse.

Lachesis

This is a useful remedy to have on hand if you're female because it treats all manner of problems caused by hormones. Not only can Lachesis support during menopause, but it also helps to lessen the physical and emotional effects of premenstrual syndrome (PMS), including mood swings, cramps, and sweet cravings. Lachesis is a great emotional healer in general and can be combined with ignitiatism to help you recover from sudden grief.

Arsenicum

Arsenicum is made from arsenic, a poisonous element, so it probably comes as no surprise that it can help you recover from another type of poisoning—food poisoning! It works best when helping your body to remove outside irritants, which is why it's also an excellent remedy for hay fever and other allergies, especially seasonal ones. People who often feel cold might find Arsenicum works especially well for them.

Lycopodium

Another useful remedy for problems of the digestive tract, lycopodium helps to soothe irritation of the stomach lining and bowel. Any problems with indigestion, excess stomach acid, a build-up of gas, and constipation are all within their wheelhouse. Lycopodium also helps to solve problems in the organs around your digestive tract including the liver.

Magnesium Phosphoricum

This is an alternative remedy for PMS problems that include sharp, stabbing cramps. If you find yourself feeling oversensitive and irritable rather than weepy and sad, Magnesium phosphoricum could be the remedy for you. It can also reduce the symptoms of other conditions that are characterized by sharp pains like neuralgia and sciatica.

Pulsatilla

Like Ayurvedic medicine, homeopathic remedies are more suited to people of specific constitutions, which is why it's always a good idea to meet with a homeopath so they can evaluate which remedies are best suited to you personally. Pulsatilla is a supportive tonic for children (and adults) who are whiny, clingy, and pale and who always seem to be suffering from a mild cough or cold. It helps to boost the body's own immune response and promote physical and emotional well-being rather than treating a specific illness.

Flower Remedies: Homeopathy for Your Emotions

The holistic philosophy that your health is split into four pillars—mental, emotional, spiritual, and physical—and, therefore, should not be treated separately is something that modern medicine is beginning to recognize. It might seem ridiculous that we're having to rediscover something that ancient civilizations took for granted, but that's just how progress works sometimes. As the medical world advanced its understanding of physical treatments, the other aspects got left behind. Over the last few decades, it's become obvious how much mental health problems can affect you physically. So the medical community has now turned its focus towards improving care in that area.

In the world of homeopathic healing, an interest in boosting emotional health has been around for nearly 100 years. Dr Edward

Bach, a homeopathic practitioner and qualified doctor from England, started developing remedies specifically to help patients cope with negative emotions in the 1930s. He believed that the body couldn't be properly healthy unless your emotions and emotional energy were in a positive place and that negative emotions actually blocked the body from healing itself. While some homeopathic remedies are designed to help with mental and emotional problems like recovering from grief, there weren't any treatments for things like loneliness, uncertainty, or fear.

Healing From Nature

Bach turned to a combination of homeopathy and herbalism to create his patented flower remedies. There are 38 in total, each one of them an incredibly gentle tincture containing the diluted essence of a plant. The remedies are grouped by their emotional effect into seven different categories, known today as:

- face your fears
- know your mind
- live the day
- reach out to others
- stand your ground
- live and let live
- find joy and hope

Bach flower remedies are designed to work slowly, so they are most beneficial when taken regularly and over time. They are sold as tinctures and can be taken as a couple of drops straight onto the tongue or added to water and sipped over the course of the day. You are even encouraged to mix the essences together to create your own personal blend because it's likely that you are feeling the effects of a few negative emotional states at once. You can find more information about the different Bach flower remedies and which ones will be able to help you by visiting their website, bachremedies.com.

Rescue Remedy

Alongside the single essence remedies, Bach created one special blend that was designed to work a little differently. His Rescue Remedy is a unique mixture of five different flower essences and should be taken as a floral first-aid remedy when you're feeling stressed or anxious. A few drops on the tongue can help to calm your nerves and relax your mind. People use it when they feel overwhelmed, like before an important meeting, an exam, or when being a parent feels too much. Rescue Remedy acts quickly and restores your emotional balance.

Holistic Herbal Healing - Review Request

Please help others who would benefit from a life of improved health by leaving this book a review.

"Sharing the gift of holistic healing with people we care about is an act of love."

People who give without expectation live longer, happier lives and feel a sense of gratitude. So together we have the opportunity to help enrich the health and lives of others..

To make that happen, I have a question for you...

Would you help someone you've never met, even if you never got credit for it?

Who is this person you ask? They are like you. Or, at least, like you used to be. Searching for guidance in improving the quality of their own health and needing help, but not sure where to look.

Our mission is to make holistic healing with nature's medicines accessible to everyone. Everything we do stems from that mission. And, the only way for us to accomplish that mission is by reaching...well...everyone.

This is where you come in. Most people do, in fact, judge a book by its cover (and its reviews). So here's my ask on behalf of a struggling person seeking better health you've never met:

Your gift costs no money, takes less than 60 seconds to make real, but can change a fellow human being's life forever. Your review might just be the encouragement they need to:

...balance mind, body and spirit.

...develop harmony and balance in their lives.

...improve the quality of their health.

..reduce reliance on conventional medications.

...open the door to positive living.

To get that 'feel good' feeling and help this person for real, all you have to do is...and it takes less than 60 seconds...to leave a review.

Scan the QR code below to leave a review:

If you feel good about helping a faceless fellow human being you are my kind of person. Welcome to the club. You're one of us.

I'm that much more excited to help you achieve a new level of health and vitality faster and easier than you can possibly imagine. You'll love the eye opening strategies I'm about to share in the coming chapters.

Thank you from the bottom of my heart. Now, back to our regularly scheduled programming.

With gratitude,

James Mercer

PS - Fun fact: If you provide something of value to another person, it makes you more valuable to them. If you'd like to share goodwill straight from another health conscious person and you believe this book will help them - send this book their way.

6. Emotional and Spiritual Healing

You could probably explain to someone what physical and mental health is, but the other two pillars of holistic healing —emotional and spiritual health—are often a little harder for people to define. Even if you think you understand the concept, putting it into words or giving tangible examples can be difficult. This is one of the reasons why these two pillars have been neglected for so long by modern medicine.

Separating emotional and mental health is probably the hardest because they both deal with feelings, emotions, and behaviors. Being mentally healthy means you have the faculties to make rational decisions, evaluate and deal with a variety of situations, and know the difference between good and bad choices. If you're suffering from poor mental health, you might act out of character or make decisions that are harmful or put you in danger.

We also recognize that there are a number of mental health disorders with specific diagnoses and treatments, including schizophrenia, generalized anxiety disorder, depression, and bipolar disorder. There aren't really any emotional health equivalents, which can make it harder to view your emotional health as suffering—if there isn't a name for it, is it really an illness?

However, all those mental health disorders existed long before they were even categorized and named. Traditionally, holistic practices have recognized emotional health issues, and although they didn't have names for them, they described them by how they appeared. So, a patient who was heartbroken might be offered rose or motherwort, and a patient who is agitated would be recommended eucalyptus.

What is Emotional Well-Being?

Emotional well-being is probably best described as the healthy processing of your emotions. It does not mean that you are happy, calm, or joyful all the time: instead, it means that you don't let your negative emotions overwhelm and control you. By constructively managing, processing, and understanding all your positive and negative emotions, you can stay in control of your behavior and navigate through daily life in a productive and enjoyable manner.

Someone whose emotional well-being is suffering will find emotions can be overwhelming, leading to an uncontrolled release of emotion in the form of crying, shouting, or hysteria. They might find it difficult to switch from one mood to another, either feeling stuck in a sad, irritable, or depressive state or being prone to mood swings that they can't control. They can also feel fatigued and find it difficult to concentrate or become agitated and anxious. Many of these symptoms are similar to those of low mental health, which is why holistic therapists are trained to not just look at symptoms but also place them into context.

Emotional Stressors

Most emotional well-being issues are caused by big changes happening in your life. Big changes, whether exciting or upsetting, bring about big emotions, and failure to deal with these in the correct way can have huge consequences. Imagine someone who finds out they're going to become a parent for the first time. They experience huge amounts of positive emotions—pride, joy, and excitement—but instead of being able to channel these emotions into a productive outlet, they become stuck, and after a few days of feeling overwhelmed, our new parents start to feel anxious, stressed and begin to struggle. They burst into tears randomly and lose their appetite. They don't understand why they're sad about something that is supposed to be exciting and worry that their friends and family will think they're acting "wrong." If this behavior continues, it could lead to strained relationships, mental health issues, and even physical problems, especially if they start acting dangerously or irrationally.

Knowing that something is going to be emotionally stressful can help you identify times to focus on your emotional health. Some typical events include:

- a new job, promotion, or pay rise
- losing your job, getting a disciplinary warning, or retiring
- changes in your romantic relationship, such as moving in together, getting engaged, getting married, breaking up, or filing for divorce
- changes to your family, such as welcoming a new child or dealing with the death of a family member
- moving house, especially if it's to a completely new area
- experiencing challenges like addiction, homelessness, pregnancy loss, or financial hardship

- unexpected periods of serious illness or a health scare, even if it turns out to be false

Help for Your Emotional Health

If you allow your emotional well-being to suffer over a prolonged period, you'll start to see an effect on your physical health. Being constantly fatigued can leave you more susceptible to illnesses, as your body won't have the energy to fight off mild viruses like a cold or a sore throat. Increased irritability and feeling angry and on edge all the time could raise your blood pressure and give you a headache.

There are herbal remedies you can take to boost your emotional health, but there are also holistic therapies and some self-help activities you can do as well. Even something simple like taking a walk in nature can be an instant mood booster and give you some much-needed space to start processing any pent-up or stagnant emotions.

Get Moving

If you're feeling low, raising your heart rate and getting your blood pumping around your body is a surefire way to make you feel better. When you feel better, you are less likely to wallow in and focus on negative emotions and start to see the positives instead. It doesn't matter if you're an exercise fan or not; there are lots of different ways to add a bit of movement to your day. Put on an upbeat song and dance in the kitchen while you're waiting for your coffee to brew or your dinner to cook. Play a game of chase with a pet or child, run laps around the garden, or lift some weights. All you need is five or ten minutes of exercise to get a boost of mood enhancing chemicals to the brain.

Relax

Low emotional health can leave you feeling anxious and plagued with intrusive thoughts that won't go away. Many of us find it difficult to switch off from our busy lives and truly find some calm and inner peace, but with a bit of practice, you can learn to turn off your worries and enjoy some emotional quiet. Take ten minutes to sit down with no distractions, close your eyes, and breathe deeply. Sip a cup of herbal tea and listen to nature sounds or relaxing music. Do a short yoga routine or some deep stretching to release tension. Take a bath and listen to a podcast or an audiobook.

Be Mindful

When your emotions are out of your control, it can feel confusing, especially if you aren't sure why. Practicing mindfulness can help you ground yourself when you feel like everything is getting away from you. It also makes you look inward and see what's really going on. Perform a body scan as described in chapter two. Think back over your day and focus on some of the moments that made you feel negative: Can you re-frame them in a more positive manner? Close your eyes and concentrate on what you can hear, smell, and feel in the room around you. Ask yourself how you are feeling and really try to identify the emotion and where it's come from.

Find the Positive and Be Grateful

It's always easier to focus on negative experiences and emotions than it is to find the positive. Something that's now being extensively recommended for mental and emotional well-being is the use of journaling to help you evaluate your experiences and find those moments of good among the bustle of the day. Each day, think of three things that made you smile and three things you are grateful for. Think about your hopes for the next day and how you can manifest them. Spread positivity to others and you'll feel it yourself: tell someone why you appreciate them, do a selfless deed, and volunteer your time for others.

Spend Time With Good People

When you're struggling with your emotions, it's tempting to wall yourself off from the world, but loneliness will only add to the problem. Identify the good people in your life: those who make you laugh, who give as well as receive, and who make you feel loved just by being there. Aim to have a meaningful conversation with someone every single day—not about work or the weather, but about how you're both feeling, what is going on in your lives, and your hopes for the future. Try to see people in person rather than only communicating over text or on a phone call. Spend time in a public place like a cafe or the cinema; just having a change of scenery can give you a much-needed lift.

Ask for Help

There's only so much you can do for yourself. If you're really struggling with your emotional help and you don't have the energy to pick yourself up, reach out to others for support. There are charity helplines with trained advisors who are happy to listen to you for as long as you want to talk. They can also point you in the direction of other organizations that could help you, like a counseling service or a peer support group. Contact your doctor and speak to them about how you're feeling, or make an appointment with a licensed therapist. If you are part of a religious group, drop in and speak to your leader or other trusted members of your faith community.

A Spiritual Connection

Spiritual health is the part most often neglected because it seems to be completely at odds with the ways of modern life. We are told to work hard and earn money to buy the newest and best items, but does this bring happiness and fulfillment? If you aren't spiritually healthy, it won't matter what car you drive, how big your house is, or how many international vacations you take each year. To truly feel inner peace and connected to a world that values you, you need to look beyond material possessions and your achievements at work.

In order to find spiritual wellness, you need to know your values: What is important to you, makes you feel complete, and feels deeply rewarding? It could be a desire to help people, for example, by volunteering for a charity, supporting your children in their studies, or caring for an elderly relative. Perhaps you feel most alive when you are creating something new, like music, a dance routine, or art. Some people feel spiritually whole when they practice their religious beliefs and are part of a wider community. There's no real right or wrong answer to how you should feel spiritually well; it's unique to each individual.

If you aren't able to spend time doing the things that make you spiritually fulfilled, you might start to feel disconnected from the world, those around you, and the life you currently lead. When you don't think you're adding value to the world, it's very difficult to find the energy or the willingness to go on because it seems like nothing matters. This sense of ennui should be a clear sign that you're focusing your efforts in the wrong place.

Someone who values helping others but cannot find the time outside of work to commit as many hours to this as they would like is going to start to feel dissatisfied with their life. The best way to re-balance their spiritual health would be to prioritize activities that align with their key values. Some ways to refocus your life around your spiritual health are

- look for a new career that directly aligns with your core values
- make a conscious effort to regularly spend your free time on a meaningful activity
- practice daily gratitude
- work on developing a more positive mindset
- spend time in nature
- develop personal rituals that connect with your spirituality

Feeling Positive

Another downside of modern society is that we are constantly being fed negative attitudes and taught to focus on what we don't have. This is great for businesses as it creates demand for their products, but it isn't a healthy state of mind to have in the long run. People nowadays are going through life constantly feeling bad that they don't have the perfect figure, the latest gadgets, or the most up-to-date home decor. Instead, you need to learn to appreciate what you have and see the many positives in your life. This positive mindset will make you feel more satisfied, more happy, and ultimately spiritually fulfilled.

Practice Self-Affirmations

These are short, positive sayings you can use throughout the day to remind yourself of the good things in your life. Some affirmations are general—"I work hard, and I deserve the praise I receive"—while others can be more specific to certain situations you're currently dealing with—"That relationship has ended because I grew and matured in a different direction, and that's okay." Repeating affirmations like these can start to rewire your brain to think more positively.

Develop a Growth Mindset

Instead of dwelling on something bad that happens, find a way to get something positive out of it. Having a growth mindset is all about looking forward and wanting to improve yourself rather than obsessing over things in the past. For example, if you are rejected for a promotion at work, don't keep replaying the interview in your head, examining everything you wish you'd done differently. Instead, ask for feedback and see this as an opportunity to grow, improve, and develop new skills that might have been lacking.

Be Kind to Yourself

You can't control everything that happens in your life, so be gentle when something goes wrong that isn't your fault. Treat yourself with the same care you would give to others in your situation. It's okay to fail, it's okay to get upset, and it's okay to feel frustrated or disappointed when things don't go the way you would have liked. Try to give yourself time to feel all these emotions and to deal with them rather than bottling them up. That might mean taking a personal day, binge-watching your favorite TV show with a tub of ice cream, and just giving yourself space to feel your emotions. You can't move forward unless you've fully processed the present.

7. Traditional Holistic Therapies

Today, traditional medicines and therapies fall under the umbrella term Complementary and Alternative Medicine (CAM). This encompasses everything that isn't a modern pharmaceutical or surgical treatment. Some practices, like osteopathy, require anyone offering these treatments to be formally trained and certified, while others, like yoga or meditation, don't. Some forms of CAM are steeped in traditions going back thousands of years and supported by vast amounts of anecdotal evidence. Others, like homeopathy, were developed much more recently.

It can be a bit of a minefield trying to navigate all the alternative therapies. How do you know which ones really work and which ones don't? Some CAMs are well-accepted in society and are often recommended by doctors to help with recovery from injuries or as a mental health treatment. However, it might surprise you to hear that there isn't always as much scientific evidence for some of these as their reputations would suggest. There is strong scientific backing for many herbal remedies, but they are still viewed as something for hippies and liberals.

At the end of the day, it should be a good thing that there are so many holistic therapies available because it gives people more choice and agency over their treatments. Most of these therapies are gentle and non-invasive, so you usually don't have anything to lose by trying them; if one doesn't help you, another might. Many doctors now practice Integrative Medicine—where they prescribe CAM alongside modern medicinal treatments (e.g., herbal remedies and acupuncture alongside chemotherapy)—because they recognize the immense benefits of taking a holistic approach to healthcare.

Alternative Systems

At one time, these alternative therapies were the main source of medical help, but they were sidelined as modern medical techniques became more advanced. The main distinction between modern and alternative medicine is in how illness and recovery are viewed: Modern medicine seeks to kill or remove the cause, whereas alternative therapies focus on helping the body heal itself. This might be through boosting its immune response with herbs, realigning its energy, or balancing *doshas*.

On your first meeting with your CAM practitioner, they will ask you about how you are feeling and why you've come to see them. They will probably probe further into your lifestyle and medical history so that they can fully understand all the stresses and aspects of your life that could be influencing your health. You might not think something is important, but to a trained holistic therapist, knowing all about your childhood, your hopes, and even your previous meals can help them make the best recommendation for your treatment.

Some CAMs involve practitioners physically manipulating your body, putting their hands on you, or using other equipment like needs, stones, and oils. This doesn't necessarily focus on the affected areas; in fact, many body manipulation therapies actually avoid them entirely. For example, reflexology involves the gentle manipulation of the feet to treat illnesses and discomfort throughout the body. Practitioners believe that each part of your foot is linked with other areas, such as your nervous system, major organs, and muscles.

Body manipulation therapies often focus on your internal energy flow and anything that is disrupting it. However, there are other CAMs that also view external energy sources as important influences on your own health. These practitioners believe that everything in the universe has an energy force, and, like the moon affecting the tides on Earth, the energies we come into contact with can affect our own life force, for good and for bad. By stimulating the flow of energy within and around your body, you can remove negative influences and help your body to rebalance.

Many CAMs also integrate healing of the mind into their treatments. Some, like meditation and hypnosis, concentrate solely on emotional and spiritual healing, while others, like yoga and Tai chi, combine these with aspects of physical and energy healing. For people struggling with the mental effects of a diagnosis, trauma, lasting injury, or long-term medication, holistic treatments like these that reinforce the connection between their mind, spirit, and body can be lifesaving.

Complementary Therapies to Try

This is by no means an exhaustive list of all the complementary and alternative therapies that are available. It is also not meant to be a list of recommended, tried-and-tested, or "proven" therapies. Instead, treat this section as an exploration of some of the more well-known or commonly practiced CAMs where you are likely to find a practitioner who is reasonably local.

Acupuncture

This therapy comes from Ancient China, and it aims to help regulate the flow of your body's life energy, known as your *chi*. This *chi* flows around your body in set pathways known as meridians. An acupuncturist will look for places where your *chi* is blocked or where its flow is sluggish, as this will be the cause of any pain and discomfort you are feeling. By inserting small, thin needles into these blocked meridians, your acupuncturist can stimulate the flow of *chi* and revitalize the areas of your body that need it most.

During a session of acupuncture, you can expect to be sitting or lying down in order to enable the acupuncturist to have free access to the site they need to treat. They will usually insert a number of needles, which might sting or pinch slightly as they go in. They might rotate the needles to encourage energy flow. Some people feel a subsequent aching at the site of the needle, like the feeling of tired muscles after a workout. The needles will typically need to stay in place for 20-60 minutes. Sometimes, the needles will be connected to a small machine that can pass a gentle electric current through them to further stimulate the flow of *chi*.

Ayurveda

Ayurveda is all about seeking balance, the balance between body, mind, and spirit, as well as a balance between different elemental influences and your body's energies. This balance doesn't mean that everything is equal. Instead, practitioners believe that you have your own unique energy fingerprint, or *prakturi* and that it is deviations from this that cause illnesses and other issues. Knowing your *prakturi* will help you identify which foods and herbs will have an affinity with you: someone with an overactive hot and dry *prakturi* could reduce it by eating foods that are naturally sweet, like wheat and fruit.

For the best results, don't just seek out Ayurvedic help when you feel unwell; this holistic system is all about maintaining health rather than the reactionary treatment of symptoms. Practitioners believe that keeping your body in balance is the best way to prevent health problems and give your body the best chance of healing. A consultation with an Ayurvedic practitioner will involve a physical examination and in-depth questioning to determine which *doshas* are dominant in your *prakturi*. This will help them advise you on ways to increase or decrease the energy flow through each *dosha*.

Traditional Chinese Medicine

Like Ayurveda, TCM believes that the key to good health is the balance of your life energy or *chi*. When this occurs, the opposing energies of yin and yang (which also have an effect on your body) are balanced too, achieving happiness and harmony. Blocked *chi* will disrupt the balance of yin and yang energies and practitioners believe that this is the cause of disease in the body. Your energies can be put out of balance by one of three things: negative energy in your environment, disrupted emotions, and bad lifestyle choices, including an unhealthy diet.

In order to restore balance, TCM practitioners will recommend a variety of treatments: herbal remedies, acupuncture, massage, nutritional therapy, exercise, and moxibustion (burning herbs close to the skin). A consultation will involve a physical exam where the TCM practitioner examines you for signs of energetic imbalance, often looking at your hair, eyes, skin, tongue, and nails, taking your pulse, and even listening to your voice. They will also ask you about your medical history, as this can give clues about your susceptibility to different illnesses, like sore throats, which will point them toward a weakness in one of your meridians.

Chiropractic

One of the most well-known alternative treatments, chiropractic was only founded in 1895, making it also one of the newest alternative treatments. The ideas behind its methods can be found in the writings of Hippocrates, who talked about a healthy spine being an important factor in maintaining good overall physical health. Chiropractors will use their hands to manually move your joints, muscles, and bones, especially those in and around your back. You will probably hear popping and cracking sounds and feel a relief of tension or pressure. This can return mobility to your back if it's been restricted by injury, stress, or trauma.

The theory behind chiropractic treatments is that a slight misalignment in your spine can pull muscles and tendons away from their optimum position and cause pain and stiffness. If you spend a lot of time bent over a computer, you might find that, after time, your neck and shoulders start to feel stiff and you have frequent headaches. Visiting a chiropractor who can release the built-up tension in your shoulder muscles should make you feel a lot better. But chiropractic isn't for everyone: If you have osteoporosis, arthritis, or a herniated disc, you should avoid this intense therapy.

At a consultation, your chiropractor will physically examine you. If you've been referred by the doctor, they might have provided x-rays or other test results that your chiropractor will use to evaluate the best course of treatment. They won't always go straight for spinal manipulation: Sometimes, they will recommend exercises, stretches, or massage instead.

Meditation

Meditation is one of the oldest forms of mental health support and dates back to more than 5000 years ago, (Peterson, 2023). Even though it had been practiced in India and China for thousands of years, meditation only really became popular in the Western world in the 1960s. However, it is now widely recognized as one of the most useful practices to help relieve stress, anxiety, and other mental health issues. Meditation is all about trying to calm and quieten your brain when thoughts become overwhelming. It does this by getting you to take a pause and just exist in the moment with your current emotions, which forces you to respond to your feelings.

There are many different types of meditation, and you can learn to do them at home or be taught by a knowledgeable practitioner. Some meditation practices ask you to focus on developing an awareness of your surroundings or your body. Others get you to visualize certain images or scenarios that are designed to be relaxing. Meditation can also be used to manifest positivity through the repetition of mantras and affirmations, either directed inwardly (cultivating a positive image of yourself) or externally (sending good thoughts to friends and family). It can take time to develop the focus needed to really benefit from meditation, but once you get the hang of it, it's the best way to manage your mental health without using medication.

Osteopathy

Often thought of as being similar to chiropractic, these two therapies do share some common values. Both believe that manipulating the body can help to restore physical wellness, but osteopathy doesn't just focus on the bones; instead, holistically treats all areas of the body, including organs and the nervous system. Osteopaths are also qualified medical doctors who can diagnose conditions that can't be treated by osteopathy, write prescriptions, and even perform surgery.

An osteopathic assessment can take up to two hours and is incredibly thorough. The osteopath will use their hands to examine any areas of pain, but then they will also watch how you move and ask you to perform some gentle exercises so they can see how your whole body responds to different stresses. When treating you, they will apply gentle pressure, resistance, and stretches to what they have identified as the problem areas. You will probably feel a little sore afterward as if you have been to an intensive session at the gym.

Because osteopaths are invested in holistic treatment, they may recommend a course of treatment alongside their sessions. This could include meditation or meditative movement like Tai chi, some herbal remedies, or prescription medication. They can also offer advice on prevention techniques so that your pain and stiffness don't return.

Reflexology

Reflexology has been recorded in ancient writings in Egypt, India, and China and has been one of the recommended treatments in TCM to help balance your *chi* for thousands of years. In the early 20th century, it was adopted by doctors in the United States, who developed it from a drug-free pain control method into the holistic therapy it is today. Practitioners use a map of the feet with different areas marked out. These areas correspond to parts of your body, and it's thought that applying pressure or stimulation to these areas can focus your body's attention on healing to where it is needed most. For example, the tips of your toes are aligned with your sinuses, so if you're struggling with an infection or a lingering cold, having your toes gently pinched will send healing energy to your sinuses and help to clear them.

There is no body manipulation involved, other than the massaging of your feet, which makes reflexology a gentle therapy that is recommended for everyone. It works particularly well on colds, infections, digestive issues, and hormonal imbalances. During a session your reflexologist will ask you what area of your wellbeing you would like to focus on in the session so they can pay attention to the right parts of your feet. Reflexologists are not diagnosticians and can only work as you direct them. You will have to lie on your back or recline in a chair so they can have access to your feet, and the session can last anywhere from 20-60 minutes. Afterward, you will feel an overwhelming sense of calm and relaxation.

Reiki

Although it is not a religion, the name reiki means "spiritually guided energy," and it is a healing method to help reduce stress and anxiety while also encouraging the patient to be more attuned to their own spiritual needs. It was founded in Japan in 1922 by Mikao Usai after a spiritual experience on Mount Kurama awakened him to the existence of an external life force energy that could be used to heal. Reiki involves the passing of hands over the patient by the practitioner, who uses their hands to direct healing energy into the patient. Reiki practitioners believe that if you have low levels of your own life force energy, it can lead to illnesses and anxiety.

During a session of reiki, as in reflexology, you'll be asked to identify any problem areas that you'd like to focus on. Treatment is given while you lie on a bed, often with low light and soothing music to encourage you to enter a deep state of relaxation. As there is no touch involved in reiki, it is suitable for people suffering from high levels of physical discomfort, such as patients receiving chemotherapy, or patients who find touch triggers traumatic memories. Reiki sessions are very relaxing and promote a sense of calm and inner peace, with some patients reporting they felt like they were in a healing trance or a pleasant meditative state.

Yoga

This ancient combination of meditation and movement came out of India, where there are several different disciplines. As a form of exercise, yoga is an effective way to increase your balance, flexibility, and core strength through the practice of different poses, or *asanas*. These are combined with breathing exercises and moments of inner reflection to create a truly holistic workout for your mind, body, and spirit. Yoga teachers are not medically trained, but they have the knowledge to help you safely adapt the *asanas* to compensate for any injuries or conditions (like arthritis) that restrict your movement.

You can practice yoga at home by following online videos or streaming a class, making it one of the more easily accessible CAMs. You can also attend classes in person at your local gym or studio. Yoga works by countering your body's stress responses and triggering your parasympathetic nervous system. This can lower your blood pressure and increase the blood flow to your organs, flooding your body with oxygen and nutrients. Regular yoga sessions can also increase the production of a number of chemicals that stimulate positive feelings in your brain, including oxytocin, serotonin, and dopamine—important hormones for preventing depression and helping you feel connected to the world around you.

Choosing the Right Practitioner

You'll have noticed that some of the CAMs described in this chapter need a medically qualified practitioner to diagnose and assess you, while others can be done without any guidance. It's important that you always do your research and make sure you're attending sessions with someone who is qualified and competent within their field. Although your doctor can refer you for chiropractic and osteopathy, you can also just make an appointment by yourself (although check with your insurance provider whether they will cover any self-referrals before you do).

When you're looking for a good local practitioner, make sure their credentials are listed on their website and check that they are registered with or licensed by an appropriate authority. Read reviews from other customers, especially those that are written on independent websites. Some CAM practitioners are able to work from home—primarily reiki masters, reflexologists, and acupuncturists—but others will operate out of clinics or therapist offices. If you don't feel valued or listened to by one practitioner, it's okay to look for another. Building a good relationship with professionals is important and you want to have confidence in someone who is treating your health.

8. Community Healing

One reason why pharmaceutical drugs have become the first choice for dealing with medical issues is that they're sold as an easy fix. Modern life is busy, and it's quicker and easier to deal with a headache by taking an aspirin than it is to fit in daily stretching and relaxation sessions, even though these would probably stop the headache from coming back. It takes a lot of effort and commitment to make permanent changes to your routine, but having the help of people around you can make a huge difference.

You might want to keep any changes you're making a secret at first, especially if they're for medical reasons and you don't want to have to start explaining your medical history to everyone. It's also completely understandable to be worried about failing, finding it too difficult, and slipping back into old routines, which is a lot easier to deal with if your friends aren't commenting on it. However, telling people that you've made the decision to change your routine and start living healthily will make the transition seem more real and can make you more determined to stick with your choices.

Making Changes Permanent

It takes a couple of weeks for new routines to feel settled, and in that time, a lot can go wrong. People often try to shake things up when they have lots of energy and motivation, but this mood doesn't always carry through. Just one day of feeling tired, stressed, or unwell can have you reaching for the comfort of old habits and having to start from scratch all over again. However, there are a few things you can do to give your new routine the best chance of succeeding, and they're all to do with proper planning.

Make a list of the things about your lifestyle that you want to change, e.g., getting more exercise, losing weight, going to bed earlier in the evening. Trying to change all of these things at one time is going to cause great upheaval and be very difficult to keep up. The best way to effect lasting change is to introduce it slowly, so look at your list and decide which new change you're going to implement first. Think about what might be the simplest but also what you're more motivated to attempt.

Next, think about how you're going to make changes to your routine that will bring you closer to your goal. If you're aiming to lose weight, are you going to change your portion size, cook from scratch more, join a supportive group, or try some low-fat recipes? Decide how to fit these changes into your existing schedule in the least-invasive manner. Choose a weight-loss group that happens at a time you can easily make, not one that has you rushing after work, as this gives you an excuse to skip it. Plan and prepare low-fat meals in advance so you don't find yourself reaching for the takeout menu when you're tired and don't have the energy to cook.

When You Hit a Problem

It's inevitable that no matter how well your new routine starts, at some point, something will happen that might throw you off track. It's important to anticipate upcoming issues and have a backup plan so you can still feel like you've achieved something. If you don't feel like doing the exercise you had planned, do something small instead, like a five-minute yoga routine or a quick dance party in the kitchen. Not only will you avoid the guilt that comes with skipping an activity, but you'll also still get a mood and energy boost, and you might find that afterward, you feel energized and ready for more.

Be gentle with yourself if things don't work out perfectly. Give yourself permission to fail and start again. One chocolate binge or decadent restaurant meal after a couple of weeks of eating well is not the end of the world; it won't undo all the progress you've already made, and it isn't a reason to give up for good. Try to keep your original motivation in mind and draw strength from it when you're finding it difficult to keep going.

Asking For Help and Getting It

Whether it's someone to exercise with who'll make sure you don't cancel plans or your partner agreeing to change their diet with you, support comes in many different forms. Most of your friends and family will probably offer you encouragement and emotional support but they may not realize some of the ways they are accidentally causing problems. For example, if you've explained to friends that you're cutting out processed foods, but then they order fast food for dinner, saying that it's "just one meal" and that it won't hurt. Even if you get a healthier option, it's not fair for you to have to sit and watch everyone else enjoy food that you've given up.

Be Specific

Explain to family and friends what changes you're making and share with them your motivations and reasons for doing so. This will help them understand your position. Don't just ask for them to support you; tell them exactly what you need them to do, e.g., don't bring certain foods into the house, don't tempt me to skip the gym, and respect my boundaries.

Use "I" statements

Try to keep the conversation focused on you and your needs rather than it becoming a list of things you're asking of others. For example, say, "I'd appreciate your support with my goal to reduce my sugar intake, so can we skip dessert?" rather than "You can't eat dessert when we go out for dinner because it's not fair to me." People are more likely to help others when they don't feel like they're being bossed around.

What to Do With Unsupportive Friends

If you know someone is going to disagree with your decisions— they think meditation is mumbo jumbo or tell you that trying to lose weight means you're against body positivity—you'll have to decide whether trying to get their support is worth it. You might find that avoiding the issue is safer than trying to address it, especially at the start of a new routine. Another option is to recruit some other friends to help support your decisions while you talk to them; there really is strength in numbers. Make it clear that you're not dismissing their opinions but that you need to do what is right for you and that you've thought long and hard about this decision.

Explaining a Medical Decision

The idea of making lifestyle changes in order to improve your health is pretty well known. You won't be the first member of your friendship group who has decided to go on a health kick, and you might even have been inspired by seeing someone else's results. It's unlikely that many of your friends will have negative opinions about your new routine if it's sensible and healthy. However, one lifestyle change that is sure to have everybody arguing is making the decision to step away from pharmaceutical medicines, especially if you have been receiving treatment for a serious condition like heart disease or diabetes.

Just because you've done your research and spoken to your doctor doesn't mean your friends will automatically be on board. They might worry that you've not made the right decision and be concerned for your health. Try not to take any questions or protests as personal attacks, and be assured that your friend's arguments are coming from a place of deep love and affection. You could point them towards resources that back up your decision or reassure them that you're working with medical professionals and everything is being carefully monitored.

It Takes a Village

As supportive as your friends might be, there are some things they will never be able to understand. Someone who's never smoked can't know the struggle of quitting, just as someone who's never had diabetes won't understand the emotional strain of balancing the condition. Thankfully, finding people who do share these issues has never been easier. The internet is full of supportive forums, online groups, and stories about people who have made the same changes that you are about to embark on. Your local area will have peer support groups that your doctor can point you toward, or you can find your people at the gym, library, or other community space.

One of the best ways to make lasting changes and new routines stick is by surrounding yourself with people who understand your journey and are willing to do it with you for the same reasons. A friend who joins you for a morning jog to be supportive is incredibly welcome, but it's not the same as having a friend who joins you because they also want to feel fitter or lose weight. If you're both working toward a common goal, you can push and motivate each other, be encouraging, and keep each other focused when times are tough.

It's been well proven that performing a task in a group or in front of an audience improves your performance (McLeod, 2023), and this isn't just true for competitive sports. People who attend weight loss groups or exercise classes are more likely to stick with their lifestyle changes and see improvements because they have other people holding them accountable and reminding them of their commitment. So, take this as a sign to reach out and find the supportive group that keeps you on the path to your ultimate health goals. Making changes is tricky, but getting encouragement and assistance from friends and family can help you through the hard part. Once your new routine is established, you'll wonder how you ever managed any other way.

9. New You, New Routine

In an ideal world, your daily routine would include activities to boost your emotional, spiritual, mental, and physical health, but the reality is that a typical workday is actually bad for your well-being in so many ways. Far too many people are stuck in a rut of getting up early, commuting to work, spending the entire day indoors (often at a desk), returning home after dark, and having to put the needs of their family or housework before their own. Sound familiar?

Creating a Holistic Home

Much of holistic medicine is about preventing issues rather than treating them. Things like eating a good diet, getting lots of rest, and spending time connecting with nature can mean you never end up needing antidepressants, counseling for stress, or weight loss supplements for your well-being. You will need to seek medical intervention for anything other than accidents and emergencies. Even chronic conditions like diabetes, asthma, and heart disease can be effectively managed with holistic lifestyle changes instead of lifelong medication.

Small Changes, Big Results

Sometimes, the changes that you need to make in your life aren't big, but they can still have a huge effect on your well-being. Modern life tries to get you to focus on achievements rather than peace by telling you that a good career, a loving family, and a secure home will all bring you happiness. However wonderful and fulfilling all these things are, they also bring greater amounts of stress and responsibility. This can put a strain on your emotional well-being and lead to both mental and physical health problems.

Dedicating just 10 minutes a day to improving your emotional well-being is all you need to help redress the balance. That's roughly the same amount of time it takes to make and drink a cup of coffee. Helpful holistic moments can be spread throughout your day, keeping you grounded and giving you time to check in with yourself and spot feelings of upset and anxiety before they become overpowering.

There's no single magic way to add holistic healing into your life, as everyone is different. Look back through some of the advice in previous chapters and identify actions that you think will have the biggest impact or be the easiest to implement. Switching your afternoon coffee for a cup of herbal tea is a great way to add a healthy tonic into your routine and you can choose whether to make it stimulating or relaxing, depending on what you need from the rest of your day.

Sample Routines

You might know exactly how you want to incorporate more holistic activities into your life, but if not, here are some examples to inspire your own changes.

In the Morning

Ayurvedic practitioners recommend waking an hour before sunrise so that you are ready to greet the energizing and warming energy from the sun. That might sound a little too early for some, but it is a good idea to leave yourself enough time in the morning to get ready without needing to rush. Set your alarm for at least an hour before you have to leave the house, and add more time if you're responsible for helping others get ready, too.

Have a glass or bottle of lemon water on your bedside table so you can rehydrate yourself as soon as you wake up. The citrus aroma is a great mood booster, and the added vitamin C can boost your immune system.

Change out of your nightclothes as soon as you get up. This can trigger an unconscious psychological change that signals you're ready to start the day. Staying in your pajamas might be comfy and cozy, but it also holds you back from feeling fully energized and awake.

Brew a cup of herbal tea instead of automatically reaching for the coffee. Reducing your caffeine intake can help reduce anxiety and help you maintain energy levels, rather than having them go up and down throughout the course of the day. If possible, drink your tea outside (or at least in front of an open window). Spend a couple of minutes enjoying the sounds and smells of nature to feed your spiritual well-being. If you don't have access to the outside, or if it's more of a concrete jungle than an exotic jungle, you can play nature sounds to simulate the experience.

Repeat some positive affirmations to put yourself in a good mood and raise your emotional energy for the day. You could do this as part of a meditation routine, accompanied by some yoga exercises, or even in front of the mirror while you're getting ready.

After Work

It's good to take some time to separate the events of the workday from the rest of your evening. Most people get home from work with several hours left in their day but don't use them efficiently because, mentally, the end of work feels like it's the end of the day. If you have a commute, you can use that time to transition into "home" mode, or if not, block out some time after work before you start any evening or family activities. Listen to a meditation that helps you reflect on your achievements during the day and leads you into the evening feeling positive; take a stimulating herbal tea or tonic to revitalize your energy levels; go for a brisk walk or have an energetic workout.

Practice gratitude. As a family (or on your own), talk to each other about your day and pick out three things that happened that you are thankful for. If someone helped make your day better, send them a message to let them know that you appreciated their contribution.

Do something creative that is just for you. Work on a personal hobby project like knitting a sweater or baking a cake, or enjoy a therapeutic adult coloring book. Most jobs don't let you tap into your creativity, so even though you might feel mentally tired at the end of the day, this part will have been under-stimulated. Being creative gives you a sense of achievement that triggers more happy hormones being sent to your brain and leaves you feeling satisfied.

Have a real conversation about something that isn't work-related. Even though you probably collaborated with other team members throughout the day, you won't have talked about anything meaningful. Your emotional health improves when you feel seen and understood, so sitting down with a friend, family member, or neighbor and talking about how you feel, what you're looking forward to, and if everything is okay is really important. Face-to-face is best, but if you can't manage that, then a video or audio call will absolutely work. You can even combine it with a cup of herbal tea or a bowl of herby soup.

Before Bed

Start your bedtime routine at least an hour before you want to be asleep. Your body and brain need time to switch off, especially if you've had a stressful day or an active evening. Don't just get straight into bed and expect to be able to fall asleep—this is how people end up lying awake with muddled thoughts keeping them up.

Try to switch off screens at least half an hour before you go to bed. Dim the lights if you can, as this will simulate the sun setting and trigger your body's production of melatonin, a hormone that helps you fall asleep.

Take a warm, relaxing bath. This is a great time to use some essential oils, as you can add them to the water or place them in a diffuser nearby. Choose something that helps to calm your mind and melt away your troubles, like lavender or cedarwood.

Start keeping a journal to track your moods and help you review your day. Journaling is becoming a popular form of self-care for emotional wellness, and there are lots of books you can buy with excellent templates and questions that prompt you to think about your daily achievements in a new way. Journaling can help you to be more positive and grateful, both of which are good for your spiritual well-being.

Try some gentle stretching or yoga before bed to release tensions that build up during the day. You can combine the movements with some calming breathwork—where you control the rhythm of your breathing to encourage mental stillness—and some affirmations.

Meditating in the evening is one of the best ways to get your brain ready for sleep. It will help you let go of any lingering thoughts and worries from the day. Visualization meditation is a good place to start—you can even listen to a guided session while you lie in bed. It doesn't matter if you fall asleep before the end of the recording; that just means it's worked!

A Holistic Environment

Where you perform your routines is as important as the routine itself. You're not going to get the best benefits from your meditation if you're surrounded by bright lights and lots of noise. You might not be able to control the volume of your neighbor's TV or the brightness of the street light, but there are some small tweaks you can make to your home that make the environment more welcoming and relaxing.

- Don't place couches or beds against walls you share with your neighbors. The sound from their side will be right on top of you and harder to ignore. Also, avoid outside walls if you're on a busy street.
- Invest in thick curtains. Not only will they block light from outside when drawn at night, but they will also muffle sounds from the street. Curtains can also add to the aesthetic of your room and make it feel more luxurious,

making it somewhere you enjoy being. However, remember to open them during the day to let as much light in as possible.

- Place scented aromatherapy candles or oil diffusers in the rooms where you spend the most time. You can use energizing oils during the day and then switch to relaxing oils in the evening. Diffusers are an easy way to gain the wonderful benefits of essential oils, and there are many different options available for purchase.

- Add plants. Not only do they increase the oxygen within your home, but they also help to connect you with nature. People with plants in their offices and homes are more productive, find it easier to relax, and feel less stressed. Just don't forget to water them.

- Remove clutter. When your surfaces are full of bits and pieces that don't belong, it can disrupt the energy in the room. A cluttered room makes it difficult to relax because your thoughts begin to pile up, too. It's immensely cathartic to cleanse your home of unwanted items, but make sure you only tackle one room at a time, or it can become overwhelming.

- Try to incorporate natural materials into your home decor. Using things from nature can help you feel more grounded and connected to the world. Wooden shelves and boxes, or stone bowls and vases, can add a lovely touch to any room.

- Choose to decorate in calming colors like pastels and earth tones. Loud, bright colors can be too energetic and they won't help when you want to switch to quieter energy at the end of the day. If you do want to use a pop of color, place it on the wall behind your bed or couch so you aren't stimulated by it when you're relaxing.

Setting Realistic Goals

Once you feel motivated to make changes, it's tempting to go all out and overhaul everything in one go. However, this is rarely practical, and if you struggle to keep everything going, you are more likely to revert to your previous habits and routines. The best way to make changes is to start slowly. This could mean changing only one thing at a time or beginning with those that take the least effort. For example, adding a few drops of lavender oil to your usual bath is a small change, but fitting in a bath when you would usually only take a shower is a much bigger effort.

Quick and Easy Wins

Changing small things around your house is a simple way to start. There's no need to spend hundreds of dollars, but purchasing a few good quality aromatherapy candles (and remembering to light them) will have an instant positive effect. You'll enjoy the benefits of the oils as they fill the room, and you'll also get a feeling of achievement and satisfaction that will make you want to do more. This comes from a surge of dopamine in your brain, and it's your body's way of encouraging you to continue with positive and helpful behavior.

Another good way to make sure your new habits stick is to connect them to things that you already do. Before you change into your pajamas, take a few minutes to stretch out with some yoga poses. It doesn't matter if this is right before bed or as soon as you get home from work, but if you keep it up, it will become a regular part of your winding down routine. You can also try saying some affirmations into the mirror after you brush your teeth, keeping a journal by your bed and writing in it once you get under the covers, and starting your evening meal with a gratitude exercise.

Making swaps or changes to your existing habits is also a great way to kick-start your new routine. Replace your coffee with herbal tea bags—you're still making your morning drink, you're just changing what's in it—and any snacks on your desk with less sugar alternatives. Stock up your kitchen's herb rack with delicious and beneficial herbs and spices, and make an effort to add them to every meal.

Thinking Long-Term

Other changes can be harder—like adding exercise to your daily routine if you're usually a couch potato—but by getting the smaller successes under your belt first, you'll be craving that satisfaction rush. If you want to make a more substantial change, like introducing 30 minutes of exercise each day or cutting out processed foods, the best way to make sure you don't give up is to start small and build up to your final goal. Adding one healthy meal a week or a ten-minute walk a day won't upset your schedule too much and will be easier for you to stick to.

You could also try giving yourself rewards for reaching certain milestones along the way. The first time you manage to exercise every day or run five miles in a week mark the occasion with a favorite treat, even if it's something unhealthy. It's important to keep yourself motivated when working on long-term goals, especially as it can take some time to see the results that you really want. This is easier to do if your goals have an emotional reason behind them; for example, losing weight and getting fitter so that you can play in the park with your children is a much stronger motivator than just wanting to drop a dress size or fit into an old pair of pants.

Sometimes, no matter how hard you try, you hit a bump in the road. Don't beat yourself up if you end up skipping a day or something happens that means you fall back into old habits. The next day is a new day, and you can start back on track. One bad day doesn't negate all the successes you had up until then, and it doesn't show a lack of commitment or that you're destined to fail, just that you're human. Long-term success is a marathon, not a sprint: there are times when you'll walk, times when you'll run, and others when you'll stop and take a break on the way to the finish line. But keep taking everything one day at a time, and eventually, you'll reach your goals.

10. The Future of Holistic Health

Medicine is coming full circle. For thousands of years, humans survived with their knowledge of plant medicines, holistic therapies, and limited surgery techniques. Then, an explosion of scientific knowledge brought a greater understanding of how disease was spread, and hundreds of new, effective treatments hit the market. But somewhere along the way, people became so focused on modern treatment methods that they forgot how important it was to look after their overall well-being.

Thankfully, traditional therapies and medical knowledge haven't been forgotten, and modern medicine is now looking at ways to use these alongside pharmaceutical and surgical treatments. With so many modern health problems caused by bad lifestyle choices, we can no longer keep throwing drugs at symptoms and expecting them to make everything better.

Integrative Medicine

The desire for more holistic treatments is hard for modern medicine to ignore. In the United States, 42% of the population already uses CAMs to supplement their healthcare. In Canada and India, it's as high as 70% (Seetharaman et al., 2021). Many insurance providers don't cover holistic treatments, but if they did, there's no doubt that the numbers in the US would be even higher. If the integrative medicine movement continues to gain momentum, we might soon see that as a reality.

Integrative medicine is the newest form of holistic healthcare, blending modern medical approaches with supplementary care from CAM therapists. Under the care of a conventional doctor, someone suffering from cancer and undergoing chemotherapy would be prescribed a number of different pharmaceutical drugs to help them cope with unpleasant side effects such as nausea, fatigue, mouth sores, and anemia. However, if they saw an integrative practitioner, they would most likely be recommended acupuncture, herbal remedies, meditation, and a nutritionist instead. These therapies have all been shown to help with the debilitating side effects of strong drugs without pumping your body full of additional chemicals.

It's not just lessening side effects where integrative medicine can be useful. Seventy-five percent of the United State's healthcare budget is spent on treatment for chronic diseases, many of which can be successfully controlled through lifestyle changes rather than medication (Seetharaman et al., 2021). Patients with cardiovascular disease, diabetes, some forms of cancer, and respiratory diseases are spending massive amounts of money—often unnecessarily—on courses of treatment that last a lifetime. Imagine how much could be saved if doctors referred people to CAM consultants rather than automatically reaching for the prescription pad.

In fact, in the future, you might find doctors who are able to write prescriptions for more than just drugs. Someone who has painful knees could be prescribed aqua fit classes to help them strengthen their muscles or a nutritionist to help them lose weight and ease the pressure on their joints. A patient with chronic anxiety could be given a prescription for acupuncture sessions and a consultation with an aromatherapist. When modern medicine fully embraces the knowledge and skills of traditional medicine, the overall health of the world is going to see a huge improvement.

New Holistic Therapies

Modern medicine isn't just seeking to integrate traditional therapies; it's actively seeking ways to improve upon them through the use of new technology. A new holistic therapy is beginning to rise in popularity, and it's called biofeedback. Biofeedback attempts to teach patients to have a greater understanding of their body's signals and give them the tools to control their involuntary reactions. This treatment can help patients better deal with stress, anxiety, and chronic pain, among other conditions.

When something scares you, your body will react in ways that get you away from the perceived danger: you'll jump backward, scream (to scare it away), your heart rate will increase, and your muscles will tense. These are all things that happen automatically, unlike when you choose to jump over an obstacle or shout to get a friend's attention. The reasoning behind biofeedback is that by understanding your body's automatic reactions, you can learn how to counter them. It's especially useful for people with conditions where medication isn't effective or there are limited treatment options. It's more than just learning to meditate or regulate your breathing because you get immediate feedback that enables you to fully personalize your actions.

During a biofeedback session, you are connected to machines by small electrodes and sensors. These measure your body's responses to stressors and will give you real-time feedback. While still connected to the biofeedback machines, a therapist will talk you through different relaxation techniques, such as progressive muscle relaxation, breathing techniques, visualization meditation, and systematic desensitization. Again, the machines will give you real time information about which of these techniques is having an effect on your body. You'll be able to see immediately how they're helping; for example, relaxing your jaw and neck muscles will reduce the pain from a tension headache. You can then try the same techniques without the machine and replicate the results every time you feel a new headache coming on.

Types of Biofeedback

There are different treatment options that are all designed to monitor and report on different problems. They can be physical—headaches, pain, issues regulating your temperature—or emotional—anxiety, panic attacks, and depression.

- Electromyogramic biofeedback (EMG) measures your muscle response and helps you identify areas of tension and injury. It can help to treat tension headaches, muscle pain, and incontinence and repair muscles that have been injured.
- Thermal biofeedback monitors the temperature of your skin. It can help you learn how to increase blood flow to parts of your body and can treat headaches, Reynaud's disease, and other temperature regulation issues.

- Electrodermal activity biofeedback (EDA) measures sweating and is linked to your body's fight or flight response. It can help with panic attacks, recovering from trauma, and severe anxiety.
- Pneumographic biofeedback gives you information about your breathing, specifically whether you're using your chest (shallow breaths) or your abdomen (deep breaths). Deep breathing is linked with increased relaxation and better sleep, and this method can help you train yourself to do it on a regular basis.
- Heart rate variability biofeedback monitors your heart rate, which can be affected by a number of different mental, emotional, and physical triggers. Learning to slow and regulate your heart rate can not only help with cardiovascular issues, it also treat mental problems like depression.

Neurofeedback

Another specific type of biofeedback, neurofeedback (EEG), measures the frequencies of different brain waves. By placing electrodes on your scalp, the machine can monitor your alpha, beta, low beta, theta, and delta waves. This is important because different brain waves trigger different states (e.g., if your theta wave levels get too high, you'll find it hard to concentrate) and are also indicative of brain injury or a neurological condition like attention deficit hyperactivity disorder (ADHD).

Once you can see your brain wave levels, you can learn to control them through different activities, and the EEG machine can show you how well it's working. Alpha brain waves can be increased by practicing meditation or taking part in high-intensity exercise. You can even find musical tracks and beats that are designed to match the frequency and wavelength of each different type of brain wave. Listening to these beats can stimulate your brain to increase a certain type of brain wave, putting you in the right state for sleeping, learning, or feeling creative.

No Need for Pharmaceuticals?

Something needs to change. Society has gone through rapid technological changes in the last 150 years, and it's causing major problems for people's well-being. As mentioned in Chapter Nine, the best way to effect lasting change is to do it slowly and in small steps, but this hasn't happened here, and we're beginning to see the damage it's causing: Neglected mental, emotional, spiritual, and physical well-being, increasing cases of chronic, manageable diseases, increasing numbers of antibiotic-resistant infections, increasing cases of mental health disorders...this list goes on. These are not signs of a society that is adapting well to its new situation.

Up till now, the main response from the medical community has been to treat any and all issues with pharmaceutical drugs. Overweight? Have an appetite suppressant. Depressed or anxious? Take an antidepressant. Diabetic? Take insulin for life. Sometimes, we forget that modern medicine is only a few hundred years old, and traditional medicine has been keeping people healthy for thousands of years. It's no surprise, then, that we're seeing a return to drug-free ways of managing illness and disorders.

With proper management, most cases of obesity, depression, and diabetes could be managed through lifestyle choices, supported, and monitored by trained professionals using modern methods. Think of the resources this would free up within hospitals: Funds and doctors would be reserved for the cases where surgery and medication were the only options, reducing wait times and making it easier for people who really need them to get an appointment with a consultant. If your first port of call for a mental health disorder was someone who would provide counseling and teach you management methods, rather than someone who wrote a prescription to suppress your symptoms, the chances of your symptoms recurring would be massively reduced.

Holistic Well-Being at Work

We're already beginning to see the huge advantages of taking a more holistic approach to well-being. Rather than being led by the medical community, the initiatives at the forefront of this revolution have come from the world of work. Employees all over the world are demanding better working conditions that are more supportive of their mental wellness—flexible hours, shorter working days, support groups, access to therapy, and benefits that promote healthy lifestyle choices. Employees who are burnt out or struggling with their mental health aren't productive and can end up costing the company a lot of money, and businesses that have started to invest in their staff's well-being have noticed huge improvements.

Once some businesses started offering wellness support, they became much more attractive to employees. In fact, a 2022 survey revealed that 81% of respondents would strongly consider how well an organization supported its employees' mental health when deciding whether or not to apply for a job there. Companies realized that if they wanted to attract the best applicants, they needed to radically overhaul their approach to employee mental and physical health.

A holistic workplace doesn't necessarily mean there are daily desk yoga sessions or free massages in the break room—although both are beneficial and some companies do offer them. Instead, it is somewhere that values the physical, mental, and emotional health of employees and demonstrates this through the benefits, workspace layout, and policies offered. Some of these include:

- The ability to take "no questions asked" vacations or mental health days. Not having to justify why you need a day for self-care makes people much more likely to take the time they need to rebalance and refocus.
- Anonymous surveys and data collection tools that let employees speak up and voice their opinions. This allows employers to spot patterns of unhappiness—for example, employees are more stressed when a project deadline is on Friday instead of midweek because they worry about delays impacting their weekends—and means they can make changes to help.
- Offering employee perks and benefits that encourage positive lifestyle changes, such as discounted gym membership, discounts at local healthy food retailers, cycle-to-work schemes, on-site fitness and wellness classes during lunch breaks, and healthy onsite catering.
- Adjusting the office layout to include plenty of natural light and open spaces where employees are encouraged to leave their desks and move around during the work day. Taking short exercise breaks, even if they're only five minutes at a time, can help you concentrate better, improve your mood, and even help you live longer.
- Running focus and support groups for different issues that encourage people to talk and share their problems. These groups can also feed back to the management and give people a chance to highlight things that are really important to them.

- Providing access to education on mental health, financial health, and physical health so that employees know how to look after themselves. Having tools like these can massively reduce stress and help people feel more in control of their lives.

Over to You

The medical community is embracing the wisdom of traditional therapies and seeing huge benefits for patients who no longer have to take cocktails of drugs to manage their health conditions. In the workplace, employers are reaping the rewards of improved productivity and employee retention by providing the holistic care that workers deserve. The last piece of the puzzle is up to you. By committing to making holistic changes at home, you can fully support every part of your health—mental, physical, spiritual, and emotional—and live your life free from pain, anxiety, and preventable medical problems.

Conclusion

It is absolutely possible to live a great life free from pain and worries and without the need for medical intervention. While there have been undeniably excellent advances in technology that have found vaccines and cures for horrible diseases, society's over-reliance on pharmaceutical drugs needs to end. Yes, medication can help make you feel more comfortable, but much of it does nothing to treat the actual cause of your pain (mental or physical). It's an easy fix, like a band-aid, that covers up the problem and makes everything seem normal.

But what does a band-aid actually do to heal a cut? Nothing; it's your own immune response that makes everything heal. In the same way, pharmaceutical drugs can mask symptoms and make it look like they've gone away, but without any input from you, once you take them away, the old issue will still be there, unchanged. This is why taking charge of your own holistic health is so impor-tant: by taking action to improve the four pillars of your well-being, you will feel more energized, less stressed, and ready to take on anything life throws at you.

See this as your personal commitment—a pact with yourself to prioritize well-being. Start with small steps, gradually weaving herbal remedies into your routines. Embrace holistic practices that resonate with you, making them a part of your day-to-day existence.

Taking Your Next Steps

Having read through this book, you should now have a good understanding of some of the principles behind different traditional therapies, and hopefully, you've identified one that you think will work for you. There's no right or wrong answer as far as alternative therapies are concerned: they speak to different people and offer solutions to different problems, so everyone's holistic journey is unique.

The first step on your holistic journey should be to find a qualified and licensed (if necessary) practitioner who can advise and guide you along the path to healing. If you're not sure where to start, try visiting a naturopath, as they are well-versed in many different CAMs and can evaluate which therapy would be most beneficial to you.

- If you're looking for general health support and an alternative to pharmaceutical medicines, herbal and homeopathic remedies can offer treatments for a wide range of symptoms, conditions, and infections, as well as providing tonics to support overall well-being. Homeopathic remedies are suitable for everyone, whereas herbal remedies can have contraindications, so make sure you read the information on each remedy carefully.

- If you want to treat chronic pain, recurring headaches, and migraines, consider beginning with acupuncture or reflexology. You can start with an initial consultation and make a treatment plan from there.
- If you have an existing injury or your problem is with your back or muscles, start by making an appointment with an osteopath or chiropractor. Your doctor might be able to recommend a local clinic, or you can search online for one in your area. These treatments are not recommended if you have limited movement or weaknesses in your bones or joints, as the treatment can be intense.
- If you are looking to improve your mental and emotional health, look into trying meditation, yoga, or tai chi. You can find some beginners sessions on the internet that are free to try at home or look for a class near you.
- For weight management or help choosing a healthy diet, get in touch with a nutritionist who will be able to put a personalized plan together for you. You can also join local groups that exercise together for encouragement and inspiration.

The Road to Lasting Improvement

Remember that it's going to take time to see the improvements that a holistic lifestyle can make to your well-being. You have to stay motivated and believe in the process because the outcome is definitely worth the effort. By taking slow steps and overhauling your old habits and routines, you'll start to see your hard work paying off over the following weeks and months.

After a couple of doses of herbal or homeopathic remedies, you should start to feel the effects.

After about a week of daily meditation, you should start to feel less stressed and anxious.

After about a month of regular yoga exercises, you should start to notice increased flexibility and energy levels.

The best way to view your progress is to keep track of how you're feeling each day. If you start to doubt the process, take a look back through your journal and you should immediately see the changes to your emotional, physical, mental, and spiritual health. This can also help you identify what has been particularly effective for you and if there's anything that hasn't quite benefited as much as you had hoped.

Remember, this journey is yours. Embrace it, adapt it, and let it flourish within you. And as you embark on this path to improved well-being, know that every step you take is a testament to your dedication to a healthier, more vibrant life.

A Final Word

Complementary therapies and medicines can be wonderful and effective tools when used correctly and safely, especially under trained professionals' guidance. However, they are not magical replacements for all forms of modern medicine—there's no herb to heal a burst appendix, and acupuncture won't repair your hernia. If you're thinking about CAM as an alternative approach to pharmaceutical medicine, please consult with your doctor first. Go into the appointment armed with your own research (from reputable sources) if that will make you more confident, and ask your doctor if an alternative treatment plan is possible. They will be able to help you integrate as much CAM into your treatment as they can, and if it can't replace what they have prescribed as the primary treatment, it will definitely be able to help support your recovery.

Heal From Within: Your Essential Guide to Natural Remedies and Holistic Medicine" - Review Request

Now you have the tools and knowledge you need to guide you forward on the journey to a healthier lifestyle so now it's time to pass on your new found knowledge and show other readers where they can find the same help.

Simply by leaving your honest opinion of this book on Amazon, you'll show other health conscious people where they can find the information they're looking for by sharing your passion for better health through holistic healing.

Thank you for your help. The benefits of holistic health are kept alive when we pass on our knowledge – and you're helping us to do just that.

Simply scan the QR code below to leave your review:

With gratitude,

James Mercer

References

Akhondzadeh, S., Noroozian, M., Mohammadi, M., Ohadinia, S., Jamshidi, A. H., & Khani, M. (2003). *Salvia officinalis extract in the treatment of patients with mild to moderate Alzheimer's disease: a double blind, randomized and placebo-controlled trial.* Journal of Clinical Pharmacy and Therapeutics, *28*(1), 53–59. https://doi.org/10.1046/j.1365-2710.2003.00463.x

Better Health Channel. (2012). *Chiropractic.* Vic.gov.au. https://www.betterhealth.vic.gov.au/health/conditionsandtreatments/chiropractic

Better Health Channel. (2017). *Immune system.* Vic.gov.au. https://www.better health.vic.gov.au/health/conditionsandtreatments/immune-system

Geddes, L. (2020). *The fever paradox.* New Scientist, 246(3277), 39–41. https://doi.org/10.1016/S0262-4079(20)30731-4

Guha, A., & Cameron, M. E. (2016). *What is the philosophy of ayurvedic medicine? | taking charge of your health & wellbeing.* Taking Charge of Your Health & Wellbeing. https://www.takingcharge.csh.umn.edu/what-philosophy-ayurvedic-medicine

Herbal Academy. (2019). *Herbal history.* https://theherbalacademy.com/herbal-history/

History of chiropractic. (n.d.). CORE Chiropractic. https://www.corechiropractic.net/articles/history-of-chiropractic/

History of osteopathy. (n.d.). St David's Osteopathic Clinic. https://www.sdos teopaths.co.uk/what-is-osteopathy/history-of-osteopathy/

How yoga works with modern medicine: Medical yoga therapy. (2022, July 1). MyYoga-Teacher. https://myyogateacher.com/articles/yoga-as-medicine#

Islam, Md. A., Haque, Md. A., Rahman, Md. A., Hossen, F., Reza, M., Barua, A., Marzan, A. A., Das, T., Kumar Baral, S., He, C., Ahmed, F., Bhattacharya, P., & Jakariya, Md. (2022). *A Review on Measures to Rejuvenate Immune System: Natural Mode of Protection Against Coronavirus Infection.* Frontiers in Immunology, 13. https://doi.org/10.3389/fimmu.2022.837290

Johns Hopkins Medicine. (2019a). *Chinese medicine.* Johns Hopkins Medicine. https://www.hopkinsmedicine.org/health/wellness-and-prevention/chinese-medicine

Johns Hopkins Medicine. (2019b). *Types of complementary and alternative medicine.* Johns Hopkins Medicine Health Library. https://www.hopkinsmedicine.org/

health/wellness-and-prevention/types-of-complementary-and-alternative-medicine

Karimi, A., Majlesi, M., & Rafieian-Kopaei, M. (2015). *Herbal versus synthetic drugs; beliefs and facts.* Journal of Nephropharmacology, *4*(1), 27–30. https://www.ncbi.nlm.nih.gov/pmc/articles/PMC5297475/

Kisling, L. A., & Stiegmann, R. A. (2020). *Alternative medicine.* PubMed; StatPearls Publishing. https://www.ncbi.nlm.nih.gov/books/NBK538520/

Making lifestyle changes that last. (2021). Apa.org. https://www.apa.org/topics/behavioral-health/healthy-lifestyle-changes

Mount Sinai. (n.d.). *Traditional Chinese medicine.* Mount Sinai Health System. https://www.mountsinai.org/health-library/treatment/traditional-chinese-medicine

Office of dietary supplements - ashwagandha: Is it helpful for stress, anxiety, or sleep? (2023, October 24). Ods.od.nih.gov. https://ods.od.nih.gov/factsheets/Ashwagandha-HealthProfessional/

Seetharaman, M., Krishnan, G., & Schneider, R. H. (2021). *The future of medicine: Frontiers in integrative health and medicine.* Medicina, *57*(12), 1303. https://doi.org/10.3390/medicina57121303

Seyedemadi, P., Rahnema, M., Bigdeli, M. R., Oryan, S., & Rafati, H. (2016). *The neuroprotective effect of rosemary (rosmarinus officinalis L.) hydro-alcoholic extract on cerebral ischemic tolerance in experimental stroke.* Iranian Journal of Pharmaceutical Research: IJPR, *15*(4), 875–883. https://pubmed.ncbi.nlm.nih.gov/28243285/

Slattery, E. (2023). *Ginger benefits.* Www.hopkinsmedicine.org. https://www.hopkinsmedicine.org/health/wellness-and-prevention/ginger-benefits

Ulliance. (n.d.). *How the future of work demands a holistic approach to mental well-being.* Blog.ulliance.com. https://blog.ulliance.com/how-the-future-of-work-demands-a-holistic-approach-to-mental-well-being

Wisdom Tree Yoga & Healing Arts, LLC. (n.d.). *Stoking Your Inner Fire: The Solar Plexus Chakra.* Wisdomtreeyoga.com. https://wisdomtreeyoga.com/news/stoking-your-inner-fire-the-solar-plexus-chakra/

What is reiki? (2014, October 15). Reiki. https://www.reiki.org/faqs/what-reiki

Royal College of Psychiatrists. (2015, April). *Herbal remedies and complementary medicines.* https://www.rcpsych.ac.uk/mental-health/treatments-and-wellbeing/complementary-and-alternative-medicines

10 top homeopathic remedies for your first aid kit. (2015, July 23). The Center for Homeopathic Education. https://chehomeopathy.com/10-top-homeopathic-remedies-for-your-first-aid-kit/

Justis, A. (2016, October 5). *How to make an herbal syrup.* Herbal Academy. https://theherbalacademy.com/blog/herbal-syrup/

Berry, J. (2017, February 9). *Cinnamon tea for soothing sore throats*. The Nerdy Farm Wife. https://thenerdyfarmwife.com/cinnamon-tea-for-soothing-sore-throats/

de Bellefonds, C. (2017, May 15). *What is capsaicin?* WebMD. https://www.webmd.com/pain-management/what-is-capsaicin

Felman, A. (2017, June 22). *Everything you need to know about osteopathy*. Www.medicalnewstoday.com. https://www.medicalnewstoday.com/articles/70381

Swift, K. (2017, September 29). *Thyme: Herb of the week*. CommonWealth Holistic Herbalism. https://commonwealthherbs.com/thyme-herb-week/

Wilson, D. R. (2017, October 30). *10 simple herbal remedies from your garden*. Healthline. https://www.healthline.com/health/herbal-remedies-from-your-garden

De Falla, K. (2018, March 26). *Capsaicin cream for joint pain*. Arthritis-Health. https://www.arthritis-health.com/treatment/medications/capsaicin-cream-joint-pain

De La Forêt, R. (2018, April 10). *Dried sage honey recipe*. Mother Earth Living. https://www.motherearthliving.com/recipes/dried-sage-honey-zm0z18mjzols/

Keatley, M. A., & Whittemore, L. L. (2018, July 25). *What is biofeedback and neurofeedback?* Www.brainline.org. https://www.brainline.org/article/what-biofeedback-and-neurofeedback

Midura, R. (2018, August 6). *Dandelion: Herb of the week*. CommonWealth Holistic Herbalism. https://commonwealthherbs.com/dandelion-herb-of-the-week/

Malhotra, A. (2018, August 30). *Why modern medicine is a major threat to public health*. The Guardian; The Guardian. https://www.theguardian.com/society/2018/aug/30/modern-medicine-major-threat-public-health

Kendle. (2018, September 14). *How to make herbal infusions & decoctions for wellness support*. Blog.mountainroseherbs.com. https://blog.mountainroseherbs.com/herbal-infusions-and-decoctions

Ashpari, Z. (2018, September 29). *The calming effects of passionflower*. Healthline. https://www.healthline.com/health/anxiety/calming-effects-of-passionflower

Steelsmith, Dr. L. (2018, October 18). *The 10 leading homeopathic remedies & their common uses*. The Upside by Vitacost.com. https://www.vitacost.com/blog/homeopathic-remedies-and-their-uses/

Gastroenterology HealthCare Associates. (2019, August 7). *6 signs your gut is unbalanced & how to fix it*. https://www.giwebmd.com/blog/2019/8/7/is-your-gut-bacteria-out-of-balance-6-signs-it-is-and-what-to-do-about-it

Raypole, C. (2019, October 28). *How to break a habit (and make it stick)*. Healthline. https://www.healthline.com/health/how-to-break-a-habit

Witkin, G. (2019, December 4). *How to ask your people for emotional support*. Www.psychologytoday.com. https://www.psychologytoday.com/gb/blog/the-chronicles-infertility/201912/how-ask-your-people-emotional-support

NHS. (2020, January 29). *Side effects - chemotherapy*. NHS. https://www.nhs.uk/conditions/chemotherapy/side-effects/

Traditional Medicinals. (2020, February 24). *Herbal basics: Tonics 101*. Www.traditionalmedicinals.com. https://www.traditionalmedicinals.com/blogs/ppj/the-basics-herbal-tonics

Rachel. (2020, March 20). *Top ten botanicals to help boost your immune system*. Wild Life Botanicals. https://wildlifebotanicals.co.uk/blogs/news/top-ten-botanicals-to-help-boost-your-immune-system

Groves, M. N. (2020, May 12). *How to make herbal tinctures*. Wintergreen Botanicals. https://wintergreenbotanicals.com/2020/05/12/tinctures/

Indigo Herbs. (2020, May 12). *Gentian benefits*. https://www.indigo-herbs.co.uk/natural-health-guide/benefits/gentian

Guts UK. (2020, May 26). *Introduction to gut bacteria*. https://gutscharity.org.uk/advice-and-information/health-and-lifestyle/introduction-to-gut-bacteria/

Wolfe, A. (2020, June 19). *Get up from your desk: 5-Minute walks are just as good for you as long ones*. The Muse. https://www.themuse.com/advice/walking-during-work-good-for-brain-body

Meda, K. (2020, July 16). *How to manipulate brain waves for a better mental state*. Www.jeffersonhealth.org. https://www.jeffersonhealth.org/your-health/living-well/how-to-manipulate-brain-waves-for-a-better-mental-state

Kluge, L. (2020, August 12). *Herbal allies for emotional resilience*. Ginger Tonic Botanicals. https://www.gingertonicbotanicals.com/blog/herbal-allies-for-emotional-resilience/

Brzeski, P. (2020, September 11). *Homeopathy: Energy - frequency - vibration*. FORM & HEAL HOMEOPATHY. https://www.formandheal.com/blog/homeopathy-energy-frequency-vibration

Parmar, R. (2020, October 12). *8 powerful ayurvedic herbs with their great benefits*. PharmEasy Blog. https://pharmeasy.in/blog/8-powerful-ayurvedic-herbs-with-their-great-benefits/

Jones, R. (2020, October 26). *Why food allergies are on the rise*. Www.bbc.com. https://www.bbc.com/future/article/20201023-food-allergies-why-nut-dairy-and-food-allergy-are-rising

Powerful herbs for emotional and spiritual healing. (2021, March 20). Original Botanica. https://originalbotanica.com/blog/best-herbs-emotional-healing

Hughes, L., & Goldberg, M. (2021, March 23). *13 ways to instantly be a more positive person*. Oprah Daily. https://www.oprahdaily.com/life/health/a25655113/how-to-be-more-positive/

Foley, M. (2021, April 30). *Echinacea: Herbal immune support* . The Alchemist's Kitchen. https://wisdom.thealchemistskitchen.com/echinacea-herbal-profile/

Sol, D. (2021, May 20). *Holistic medicine: A guide for beginners*. Pacific College.

https://www.pacificcollege.edu/news/blog/2021/05/20/holistic-medicine-guide-for-beginners

Burgess, L. (2021, June 17). *7 herbs to support digestive concerns.* Www.endeavour.edu.au. https://www.endeavour.edu.au/about-us/blog/7-herbs-support-digestive-concerns/

Admin. (2021, August 24). *Ayurveda: A brief introduction & guide.* The Ayurvedic Institute. https://ayurveda.com/ayurveda-a-brief-introduction-and-guide/

What is reiki, and does it really work? (2021, August 29). Cleveland Clinic. https://health.clevelandclinic.org/reiki

Team Tony. (2021, September 29). *The keys to spiritual wellness.* Tonyrobbins.com. https://www.tonyrobbins.com/health-vitality/the-keys-to-spiritual-wellness/

Chanel, A. (2021, October 22). *4 pillars of holistic health and wellness and how to harmonize them.* YouAligned™. https://youaligned.com/wellness/holistic-health-and-wellness-pillars/

Medline Plus. (2021, October 25). *Clove: MedlinePlus supplements.* https://medlineplus.gov/druginfo/natural/251.html

Aspell, N. (2021, November 5). *Lavender oil and sleep: Why it helps and how to use it.* Lavender by the Bay. https://lavenderbythebay.com/blogs/lavender-by-the-bay/lavender-and-sleep

Mayo Clinic. (2022, January 27). *11 alternative cancer treatments to consider.* Mayo Clinic. https://www.mayoclinic.org/tests-procedures/cancer-treatment/in-depth/cancer-treatment/art-20047246

Saleh, N. (2022, March 29). *Design a holistic health routine.* Spirit of Lotus. https://www.spiritoflotus.com/post/design-a-holistic-health-routine

Masterclass. (2022, April 6). *How to make dandelion tea: 3 types of dandelion tea.* https://www.masterclass.com/articles/how-to-make-dandelion-tea#2btaZpRZX8GeWiBjCDN0bT

Sissons, B. (2022, April 27). *What is emotional health and well-being.* Www.medical-newstoday.com. https://www.medicalnewstoday.com/articles/emotional-well-being

Beavan, R. (2022, June). *Simple motivation tricks: How to stick to your health goals.* Www.bhf.org.uk. https://www.bhf.org.uk/informationsupport/heart-matters-magazine/wellbeing/how-to-motivate-yourself-to-get-healthy

Larian, B. (2022, June 23). *Our favorite herbs for pain relief and inflammation.* Mdbiowellness. https://www.mdbiowellness.com/blogs/doctors-desk/our-favorite-herbs-for-pain-relief-and-inflammation

Villacorta, C. (2022, July 6). *The best homeopathic remedies to build your home kit.* Cristina Villacorta. https://cristinavillacorta.com/blog/10-top-homeopathic-remedies-for-your-first-aid-kit/

Reflexology: What it is, and does it work? (2022, August 29). Cleveland Clinic. https://

health.clevelandclinic.org/reflexology

WTHN. (2022, September 29). *Traditional chinese medicine herbs list to improve overall health.* https://wthn.com/blogs/wthnside-out/traditional-chinese-medicine-herbs-liste.

Watson, S. (2022, November 12). *Overview of Biofeedback.* WebMD. https://www.webmd.com/pain-management/biofeedback-therapy-uses-benefits

Griffin, R. M. (2022, November 29). *Ashwagandha.* WebMD. https://www.webmd.com/diet/supplement-guide-ashwagandha

Turner, K. (2022, December 6). *5 fundamental steps for achieving unity of mind, body and spirit - alleviant integrated mental health.* Alleviant. https://alleviant.com/5-fundamental-steps-for-achieving-unity-mind-body-spirit/

Brown, M.-E. (2022, December 15). *Turmeric benefits.* Www.hopkinsmedicine.org. https://www.hopkinsmedicine.org/health/wellness-and-prevention/turmeric-benefits

IQVIA. (2023, January 18). *The global use of medicines 2023.* Www.iqvia.com. https://www.iqvia.com/insights/the-iqvia-institute/reports-and-publications/reports/the-global-use-of-medicines-2023

Difference between mental and emotional health. (2023, February 22). Mindful Health Solutions. https://mindfulhealthsolutions.com/difference-between-mental-and-emotional-health/

Horstman, E. (2023, February 6). *A health coach shares her own energizing morning routine—and it's so achievable.* Camille Styles. https://camillestyles.com/wellness/holistic-rituals/

Raman, R. (2023, February 15). *12 health benefits and uses of sage.* Healthline; Healthline Media. https://www.healthline.com/nutrition/sage

Mary Jo DiLonardo. (2023, February 21). *What are Bach flower remedies?* WebMD. https://www.webmd.com/vitamins-and-supplements/bach-flower-remedies

Atlas, Z. (2023, May 19). *How to talk to friends and family about new eating habits.* Levels. https://www.levelshealth.com/blog/how-to-talk-to-friends-and-family-about-new-eating-habits

Lubeck, B. (2023, May 23). *Fennel and fennel seeds: a look at the benefits.* Verywell Health. https://www.verywellhealth.com/fennel-and-fennel-seeds-benefits-uses-and-more-7495392

Lana. (2023, June 30). *Best examples: Holistic house and holistic interior design.* Dressarte Paris. https://www.dressarteparis.com/best-examples-holistic-house-and-holistic-interior-design/

McKeown, J. (2023, July 10). *Schisandra: An herb for all reasons and all seasons (of life).* WishGarden Herbs. https://www.wishgardenherbs.com/blogs/wishgarden/schisandra-an-herb-for-all-reasons-and-all-seasons-of-life

Timmons, G. (2023, August 9). *Hippocrates - quotes, oath & medicine*. Biography. https://www.biography.com/scholars-educators/hippocrates

Centers for Disease Control and Prevention. (2023, August 23). *Tips to improve your emotional well-being*. Www.cdc.gov. https://www.cdc.gov/howrightnow/wellbeing/index.html

McLeod, S. (2023, October 5). *Social facilitation theory in psychology*. Simplypsychology.org. https://www.simplypsychology.org/Social-Facilitation.html

Marks, H. (2023, October 8). *Stress symptoms*. WebMD. https://www.webmd.com/balance/stress-management/stress-symptoms-effects_of-stress-on-the-body

Covington, L. (2023, October 11). *Stop wasting herbs—here are the best ways to dry them*. The Spruce Eats. https://www.thespruceeats.com/harvesting-and-drying-leafy-herbs-1327541

Season Herbs. (2023, October 25). *How to make thyme tea and its benefits*. https://seasonherbs.co.uk/blogs/recipes/how-to-make-thyme-tea

Nordqvist, J. (2023, November 8). *Everything you need to know about rosemary*. Www.medicalnewstoday.com. https://www.medicalnewstoday.com/articles/266370

Kubala, J. (2023, November 14). *What is valerian root?* Health. https://www.health.com/valerian-root-benefits-7094035

Peterson, T. J. (2023, November 29). *Meditation: Benefits, how it works, & exercises to try*. Choosing Therapy. https://www.choosingtherapy.com/meditation/

Millstine, D. (2023, December). *Homeopathy*. MSD Manual. https://www.msdmanuals.com/en-gb/professional/special-subjects/integrative,-complementary,-and-alternative-medicine/homeopathy

Brazier, Y. (2023, December 7). *How does acupuncture work?* Www.medicalnewstoday.com. https://www.medicalnewstoday.com/articles/156488

Pacchioli, L. (2024, January 5). *Secrets of chamomile in the treatment of digestive disorders*. NATURVEDA Plantes et Santé. https://naturveda.fr/en/blogs/actus-sante/les-secrets-de-la-camomille-dans-le-traitement-des-troubles-digestifs

Homeopathy uses and evidence base. (2024, January 15). Www.nhsinform.scot. https://www.nhsinform.scot/tests-and-treatments/medicines-and-medical-aids/complementary-medicine/homeopathy/

Mayo Clinic. (2024, January 16). *Integrative medicine and health - overview*. Mayo Clinic. https://www.mayoclinic.org/departments-centers/integrative-medicine-health/sections/overview/ovc-20464567

Tazmin, L. (1 C.E., November 30). *Holistic living: The daily routine in ayurveda*. Peaceful Dumpling. https://www.peacefuldumpling.com/holistic-living-the-daily-routine-in-ayurveda

Made in the USA
Coppell, TX
22 November 2024

40794823R00083